10-Day Sugar Detox Diet:

Smash Your Addiction and Cravings! Lose Weight! Includes 10 Day Meal Plan and 30 Savory Recipes.

By Francesca DiMarco

First Printing: 2015
Bright Ideas Editorial
PO Box 4095
Crested Butte, CO 81224
http://brightideaseditoria.com/

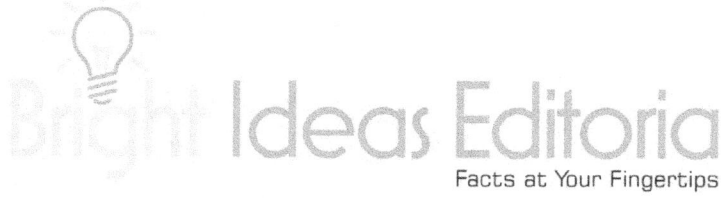

Disclaimer

Although the author and publisher have made every effort to ensure that the information in this book was correct at press time, the author and publisher do not assume and hereby disclaim any liability to any party for any loss, damage, or disruption caused by errors or omissions, whether such errors or omissions result from negligence, accident, or any other cause.

This book is not intended as a substitute for the medical advice of physicians. The reader should regularly consult a physician in matters relating to his/her health and particularly with respect to any symptoms that may require diagnosis or medical attention.

FREE DOWNLOAD

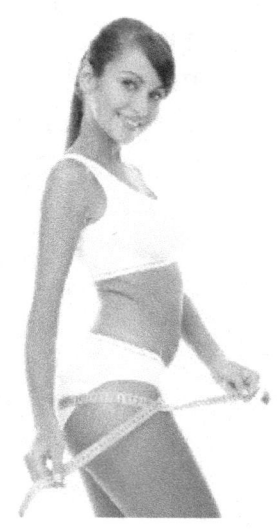

As a thank you for purchasing this book, I've created a free report full of weight loss hacks just for you!

TOP 10 WEIGHT LOSS HACKS - NO

DIETING ALLOWED!!!

"Free Report Reveals...The top 10 (ridiculously easy) weight loss hacks (Hint: You'll never believe #7)"

You can download the free report at
https://editoria.leadpages.co/weightlosshacks/

Table of Contents

Introduction

"Every form of addiction is bad, no matter whether the narcotic be alcohol or morphine or idealism."
Carl Jung, Memories, Dreams, Quotations

Growing up, my father used to say that it was harder to quit sugar than heroin. He was a picky eater with a horrible diet and was always trying to lose weight. When I was a teenager and finally understood what he meant, I wondered if my not-so-straight-laced father had a past more checkered than the cab he drove for extra cash. These days I'm *pretty sure* he was just quoting some statistic he'd heard. But the claim is intriguing and demands a closer look.

How addictive is sugar?

If you type sugar addiction into Google, you'll see hundreds of thousands of articles about a 2013 study done at Connecticut College involving rats, Oreos, cocaine and morphine. [1, 2] The students and faculty conducting the research gave the rats a choice between Oreo cookies and rice cakes, and not surprisingly, the rodents went for the cookies (and ate the white centers first). They gave another group of rats a choice between a saline injection, and a morphine or cocaine injection, and the animals went overwhelmingly for the drugs. So far no surprises. The big deal about the study was that when the researchers compared the brains of the Oreo rats and the junkie rats, they found that the high-fat/high sugar cookies activated more neurons in the brain's pleasure center than the narcotics did.

Some headlines about the study screamed "Oreos more addictive than cocaine!" That is a pretty simplistic interpretation, according to Edythe London, Ph.D., a researcher who studies the biology of addiction. She says that in order to really compare the addictiveness of the two, researchers would need to measure how many times a rat was willing to press a lever to get the substances to measure how hard they would work for it. [3] Or see if they would do little rat pole dances in a thong.

But an earlier study conducted in 2007 seems to prove overwhelmingly that rats, at least, prefer intensely sweet stuff *even to* cocaine. Researchers gave rats a free taste of super sweetened water and of cocaine, and then they showed them how to get more by pressing a lever. But the rats could only pick one. Ninety-four percent of the rats chose the sweet water, over and over. Researchers tested both sucrose, a natural sugar, and saccharin, an artificial zero-calorie sweetener, and the results were the same. Even more interesting, the researchers tried it again with rats who already had a cocaine addiction, and the addict rats still preferred the sweet water, even when the cocaine doses were increased.[4]

Does this prove that sugar is addictive? The American Psychiatric Association defines substance abuse as the presence of 2-3 of the following 11 symptoms:[5]

1. *Taking more of it than you had planned*
2. *Having trouble cutting down or stopping its use*
3. *Spending large amounts of time obtaining, using, or recovering from it*
4. *Craving it*
5. *Neglecting work, school, or home life because of it*
6. *Using it even after it is clear that relationships are suffering because of it*
7. *Avoiding work, social or family events that you would normally attend because of it*

8. Using it repeatedly even when it puts you in dangerous situations

9. Using it when you know it can make a physical or mental problem worse

10. Needing more and more of it over time to get the same effect

11. Experiencing withdrawal symptoms that go away when you take it again

When I get the image of a guy in a black beanie leaning against a brick wall whispering, "Psssst. Got your Double Stuf," out of my head, the above list gives me pause. Eating six brownies at a go, craving sweets, baking cookies even when I know I'm at risk for heart disease and diabetes. Is sugar substance abuse really a thing?

Yes, yes, and YES scientists are beginning to agree.[6] Not only does it satisfy the above criteria because of bingeing, withdrawal, craving, and increased tolerance, but it meets the definition for neurochemical reasons as well. According to neuroscientist Nicole Avena from Columbia University, too much sugar too often sends our levels of dopamine, a feel-good reward that our bodies produce, out of control (but not as much as heroine, she is quick to point out).[7] Sugar not only tastes good, it feels good, and the more we have, the better it gets. Unfortunately, the same cannot be said for broccoli, which is why no one has a green vegetable addiction.

Scientists think that the reason we react so strongly to sugar is because our brains haven't evolved to recognized processed foods yet. Sugar was first refined around the 6th century B.C., which, on an evolutionary time frame, was about 14 minutes ago.[8] Until that time, sweet tastes came only from natural sugars like those in fruits and vegetables, which signaled good things like quick energy to run from that saber-tooth tiger.[9] We just haven't have time to recognize that processed sugar now brings about bad things like heart disease and diabetes.

Does this mean we should avoid sugar all together? No, experts say. In fact, your *brain needs sugar*. Brain cells use a form of sugar called glucose exclusively as a fuel source, and they require a steady supply from your blood stream.[10] But those same experts say that we do need to moderate our sugar intake. When sugar is under control, we don't get the same dopamine spike that happens when we abuse it. Which begs the question, how much sugar should we consume?

Experts say that women should consume 6 teaspoons or less of *added* sugar a day (24 grams), and men should eat less than 9 teaspoons (36 grams).[11] That averages out to somewhere between 18 to 27 pounds of added sugar per year. Estimates for how much added sugar the average American actually consumes a year are all over the map. I've seen figures from 60 pounds to 250 pounds, which means that we each consume somewhere between the mass of an average eight-year-old child and an Ikea sofa just in added sugar.

The excess of sugar causes obesity, which in turn leads to heart disease, type 2 diabetes, premature aging and a host of other preventable diseases and health conditions.

The goal of this book is to help you to move from a place where your body is craving sugar and rewarding you inordinately for eating it, to a place where you can enjoy an occasional treat but are not a slave to it. Breaking your sugar addiction will allow you to establish a nutritious eating plan, lose weight, and live much healthier. It's not going to be easy (insert your own cliché). But after you do it, you'll feel a whole lot better.

Before we get into how to break your sugar addiction, we need to establish a definition as to what sugar is. The next chapter looks at the many forms of sugar and why your body doesn't treat them all the same.

Chapter One: What is Sugar and How Do You Use it?

"Of some delights, I believe, sir, a little goes a long way."

Elizabeth Bennet in Pride & Prejudice, screen adaptation by Andrew Davies

When my daughter was four, the dentist asked me, in that deep, I'm-going-to-judge-your-parenting-abilities-and-find-them-wanting voice, how much fruit juice she drank. "Almost none!" I told him because I was an awesome nutrition conscience mom.

"How about milk?" He asked.

"Oh, she drinks lots of milk! Good for strong bones and teeth!" I may have actually patted myself on the back.

"Does she brush her teeth every time she drinks milk?" Wait, what?

"Nooooooo. But-she-brushes-her-teeth-twice-a-day-and-we're-really-good-about-it." I said.

"Did you know that a glass of milk has as much sugar as a glass of juice? And it sticks right to your teeth." Huh? Milk has sugar? No, no, no, no, no! Everyone knows that milk has protein, and vitamins A & D, and it gives you a shiny coat, and it absolutely only has sugar when you put chocolate in it or dump it on one of those sugary cereals or something.

To prove his point, the dentist-who-I-was-now-sure-was-a-quack pointed to my precious daughter's x-rays and pretended he could see a cavity.

When I got home I researched the "doctor's" purported "facts", and it turns out that he was right. Kind of. It depends widely on which type of juice, of course. Milk has half the sugar of apple juice, twice as much as orange juice. Because lactose is sugar.

What, exactly, is sugar?

In biochemistry, the Latin suffix 'ose', meaning 'full of', is used to name sugars. Sucrose, fructose, glucose, amylose, dextrose, maltose, galactose, and lactose are all sugars. But they are not the only sugars. Honey, agave nectar, muscovado, treacle, molasses, diastatic malt, caramel, dextran, diatase, and anything with the word 'syrup' or 'sugar' in the name are also sugars. If so many different substances are all considered sugars, what do they have in common?

Carbohydrates
Sugar is a simple, water soluble carbohydrate. Carbohydrates are molecules made up of carbon, hydrogen, and oxygen atoms and are one of the three macronutrient food groups, along with fat and protein. Carbohydrates come from plant and dairy products. Simple carbohydrates, or sugars, dissolve in water, and are made up of only one or two carbohydrate molecules. Your body can pull them apart and digest them in a snap, which is why they provide quick energy.

Complex carbohydrates, like fiber and starch, are longer,

more intricate sugar chains (think thousands of molecules instead of one or two) that your body has to work harder to break apart to get at the energy. Your body digests starch carbs more slowly than simple sugar, so the sugar spike is less. The more refined the carbohydrate, like white flour instead of whole wheat, the easier it is for the body to convert the chain into simple sugar (and the fewer micronutrients that remain).

Fiber is different. Your body doesn't make the right enzymes to dissolve the links between the sugar molecules in fiber, so it passes on through.[12] This is why people who count carbs are allowed to subtract the grams of fiber from the total carbohydrates. But even though your body doesn't get any energy from fiber, fiber is still very useful. It takes up a lot of room in your belly so it makes you feel full longer. It slows down digestion, further reducing sugar spikes. It reduces inflammation in the gut. It prevents and cures constipation, and even reduces LDL (L for lousy) cholesterol.[13]

What is the Glycemic Index?

People often reference the Glycemic Index when talking about carbs. The Glycemic Index is a quick-and-dirty scale that tells you how fast your body converts a carbohydrate into usable sugar, usually glucose. Higher numbers are converted more rapidly; lower glycemic numbers are slower to convert. It is based on the conversion rate of pure glucose, which has a Glycemic Index of 100. The lower the number is, the better it is, usually, but there are always other factors to consider.

Glycemic Load is the Glycemic Index of a food multiplied by the number of carbohydrate units in a serving.

The way your body uses sugar depends on whether it breaks down into glucose or fructose. This is a simplified explanation of a very complicated process.

When you consume sugar or starch, your body breaks down most of the different forms into glucose during digestion.[14] I visualize a bunch of different kids getting the same haircut and school uniform on the first day of the year. The glucose is released into the bloodstream like a pack of excited children running around on the playground. Your pancreas gets notified to send out insulin to manage it. Insulin is a hormone that, like a brave school teacher with a set of keys, opens the doors to many types of cells and allows the sugar to come in and get to work.[15] Twenty percent of the glucose goes to your brain, which is why you can't think well when you have low blood sugar.[16] If there is more sugar in your body than you have need of, the insulin walks it single file without talking down to your liver, where it gets sent to time out (converted to glycogen), and waits to be used in the liver or muscles, or is converted to fat (triglycerides) and stuck somewhere like your belly.[17,18]

This is why it is so important to give your body sugar it can process over time instead of all at once. When those high-spirited sugar nutrients in the blood gets so out of control that they stop responding to the wise insulin (known as insulin resistance), or the body can't produce enough insulin to manage all the sugar, the sugar stays in the bloodstream, becoming little sugar hooligans which begin to vandalize your body.[19] Picture the word 'diabetes' in red spray paint.

Fructose, however, requires extra processing. It travels

through the gut, and into a bloodstream that is sent directly to the liver. It doesn't get to run wild and free in the body, and it takes more time to metabolize than glucose does. This is why misguided (or deceitful) proponents praise fructose for having a low Glycemic Index. It also tastes sweeter on the tongue than glucose does. In the liver, enough is converted to replace the glycogen in the liver *but not the muscles*, and this is critical.[20] Once the glycogen in the liver is sufficient, the liver starts converting the fructose to triglycerides. So anything more than 'just enough' fructose turns into fat.

If fructose were a character in a Jane Austen novel, it would be Mr. Wickham from *Pride and Prejudice*. It has all the appearance of goodness, coming from natural sources like fruit and honey. It is exceptionally sweet and easy to fall in love with. But it can behave most villainously. An excess of fructose over time can lead to weight gain and insulin resistance.[21] These can contribute to heart disease and diabetes among other health conditions. A prolonged excess of fructose can also overload the liver and keep it from doing other jobs, like removing uric acid, a by-product from protein metabolism. When uric acid crystalizes on the joints, it leads to painful gout. Too much fructose also encourages wrinkles.[22] Seriously. Fructose is the bad boy of the sugar world.

Now that we've looked at what sugar is and what it does for the body, it is time to decode the different names for sugar.

Chapter Two: The Many Names of Sugar

"What's in a name? that which we call a rose

By any other name would smell as sweet;"

William Shakespeare, Romeo and Juliet

In the last chapter, we defined sugar as a basic building block of carbohydrates. We determined that carbohydrates break down into monosaccharides, or single molecule sugars, during digestion, and that the body processes the monosaccharides glucose and fructose differently. So it would seem important, then, to know what basic sugars the different sweeteners break down into so that you can choose your sugar wisely.

The terms natural and refined sugar are tossed about quite a bit. All sugars start out from natural sources, of course. Sugars are produced by plants and are present in dairy products. The level of processing that occurs before you consume the sugar should be the determination as to whether the sugar is considered 'natural' or 'refined'. The sugar in an apple is clearly natural. The white sugar in a cube is clearly refined. But not everything is so easy to categorize.

Think about the term 'natural blond' for a second. A natural blond would seem to be a person whose hair is genetically a light color. But when a person's hair turns light as a byproduct of spending time in salt water and the sun, are they a natural blond? After all, they achieved their color naturally. What about someone who purposefully uses lemon juice and sunlight to lighten their hair? Lemon juice and sunlight are natural and pure, even if the change was calculated. Does motive play a part as to whether something is natural? What about someone who uses peroxide? Hydrogen peroxide can be found (in trace amounts) in rain and snow. It exists in a natural form, even if the substance in that particular bottle was synthesized in a factory. What if you add a little color back when you start going grey? Just where to draw the line between a natural and a bottle blond isn't easy. Especially when advertisers get involved.

But the question we haven't asked yet, is, does it matter? Is it important if hair color came from your parents or your hairdresser? Regardless of the amount of processing, if done well, the hair color is perceived the same by a casual observer. It could be argued that treated hair might be less healthy. The chemical processing might have stripped away some of its natural vitality. But what if the unprocessed hair hasn't been well cared for? What if it is weak and full of split ends? And what if the treated hair has been fortified. Who can say which is better? Who can say which is healthier?

The same can be said for sugar. Many of the various 'natural' sugars aren't as pure as manufacturers would have us believe. And some of the processed sugars aren't as terrible. Here is a closer look at natural and processed sugars.

Natural Sugar

Sugar is naturally found in plants, honey, and dairy products. From the names, it seems like fruits would have fructose, and sugarcane would have sucrose, but the reality is much more complicated. Plants, like fruits and vegetables, and honey all have fructose, glucose, and sucrose. Sucrose is a disaccharide that has one molecule each of fructose and glucose bonded together. Milk has glucose, galactose, and lactose (which is both glucose and galactose bonded together). Dextrose is the same as natural glucose. Glucose (dextrose), galactose, and fructose are all monosaccharides, which are the simplest sugar building blocks and have only one molecule. That is why the body can use them so easily. Fructose tastes sweeter on the tongue than does glucose or galactose.

Lactose and sucrose are disaccharides, which have two molecules that the digestive process can easily strip apart. Maltose is also a disaccharide and has two glucose units. Starch and fiber are polysaccharides, which have lots of molecules. As said previously, it takes much more work for your body to break starch apart into usable sugars, and it can't break down fiber.

The nice thing about the simple sugars found in fruits and vegetables is that they are accompanied by complex sugars like fiber, and small amounts of protein and fat, as well as vitamins and minerals. The simple sugars in milk also hang out with protein, fat, and micronutrients. The gut takes longer to process the complex carbs, protein, and fat, so you feel full longer and get a slow release of energy along with the quick release from the sugar.[23] The sugars aren't as highly concentrated in many natural foods as in processed ones, so you are consuming only moderate amounts of simple sugars, and getting healthy benefits along with the energy.

There are caveats, though. Once the sugar is in your belly, your body distinguishes no difference between the glucose and fructose from an apple than from an Oreo. If you consume excessive sugar from fruit, your body is at just as much risk as it is from too many cookies. It is harder to overdose on sugar from fruit, though because the fiber in whole fruits fills you up. But it becomes easier when you remove the fiber. This is why juice is such a concern among pediatricians (and dentists).

Is fruit juice a natural or a bottle blond? It comes from a natural source, but it is processed, at least minimally (and sometimes a lot more) to extract the juice. It is used as a 'natural' sweetener, like honey, and like honey they both have glucose and fructose, and the higher the concentration of fructose they have, the sweeter they are. Also like honey, fruit juice can have trace amounts of micronutrients and fiber. And like fruit juice, honey undergoes processing before you buy it in the supermarket. Most honey is pasteurized to remove the crystals and yeast spores, which can reduce the health benefits.[24] Both honey and fruit juice are sweeter than table sugar and have more calories, so when used as a substitute for table sugar, you need to use less.

And what about the most misunderstood 'natural' sugar of all, agave nectar?

Agave nectar is to natural sugar what Marilyn Monroe was to natural blonds. Agave nectar comes from the same plant as tequila. Due to slick marketing, it is now often viewed as a healthy alternative to sugar. Consider, though that there is no spigot on an agave plant. Agave needs to be highly processed before it turns into agave nectar or syrup, so you aren't getting additional micronutrients or fiber. Due to the high concentration of sweet fructose, agave enthusiasts tout that you can substitute less agave for refined sugar. Agave syrup has 50% more calories than table sugar, 60 per teaspoon compared to 40, so to reap any benefits, you need to use 1/3 less. Advocates also say it is lower on the glycemic index than table sugar.[25] Fair enough, but that isn't a license to use it without restraint. Remember that fructose turns to fat faster than any other sugar.[26]

When it comes right down to it, except for the sugar found in whole foods, all natural sugars are refined to a certain extent. Now, though, let's look at the really refined sugars.

Refined Sugar

Humans began refining sugar before Buddha attained enlightenment or Confucius wrote any fortune cookies. We've gotten really good at it.

Sugars are produced by plants during the process of photosynthesis. Sugarcane is used to produce about three-quarters of the world's sugar[27] (we'll get to corn syrup in a minute). Sugar beets are used to make the rest.

Sugarcanes are grown, harvested, cleaned, and then shredded and compressed to extract all the juice. The cane juice is then clarified and evaporated until it is in syrup form. Following this, it is crystalized and the crystals are separated from the molasses. When it is dry, it takes the form of raw sugar, and then it is refined into the sugar that is popularly consumed.[28] Refined sugar is mostly sucrose, which is one molecule each of glucose and fructose bonded together.

Sugar beets are processed by slicing and boiling the beetroots. The sugar dissolves into the water. The pulp is used for animal feed, and the remaining juice is crystalized and the sugar is separated from the molasses.[29] Sugar from beets and cane is identical.

Some of the most popular forms of sugar are[30]:

White sugar (also known as regular sugar, extra fine sugar or fine sugar). This is the most common household sugar, used in baking and morning coffee.

Fruit Sugar - This has a larger percentage of fructose, so it is sweeter than white sugar. It has crystals which are finer than white sugar, and it is used in puddings, powdered drinks, and gelatin.

Castor Sugar - This is the finest of all white sugar. It is mainly used in baking, and for sweetening cold drinks as it dissolves easily.

Confectioners' Sugar - This is ground white sugar with a little corn starch. It is used in whipping cream and icing.

Brown Sugar (Dark and Light) - Sugar, which has been refined, and then has molasses added back in. The darker it is, the more molasses it has. It contains more moisture than white sugars. Because brown sugar has more plant material left in it, it may contain slightly more antioxidants, vitamins, and minerals, but has more or less the same calorie content as white sugar.

Muscavado Sugar - A stickier stronger flavored form of dark brown sugar.

Demerara Sugar – Called 'raw sugar' in the US, brown sugar that has less molasses.

Liquid sugars are simply white sugars which have been dissolved in water.

And then there is corn syrup.

Corn sugars have been around since the late nineteenth-century. Corn starch is refined into pure glucose, which, if you have been paying attention, isn't as sweet as the half glucose/half fructose table sugar, but is easier for your body to use.

It wasn't until the 1950s that the liquid corn syrup was developed, and it had a number of advantages over sugar. It was less expensive to produce, and the liquid form made it easier to incorporate into food products. But it still wasn't as sweet.

In the late 1960s, Japanese scientists figured out how to convert some of the glucose in corn syrup into fructose, creating High Fructose Corn Syrup.[31] If you were to remove the water from HFCS, the remaining mixture would be either 55% fructose, used in soft drinks, or 42% fructose, which is used in most other food products.[32] This isn't radically different that the fructose content found in table sugar. So what, then, is the big deal about high fructose corn syrup and obesity?

One reason, according to Barry Popkin, Ph.D., nutrition professor at the University of North Carolina, is that we consume so much of it.[33] Because it is so easy to add HFCS to food products, manufacturers add it to everything. Food products are competitive, and producers found that adding a little bit of sweetener enhanced the flavor of everything from salad dressing to vegetable soup.[34] By sweetening everything, food companies gradually raised our tolerance for sweet tastes, and now many foods, like tomato sauce, just don't taste right without it.

Other objections to HFCS are that companies that make it are so secretive, we don't really know what is in it, according to Dr. Mark Hyman, MD. It is so processed that it contains mercury and other contaminants, he says.[35] He also says that our bodies do not process sucrose and HFCS in identical ways. The glucose and fructose in HFCS are not bonded together the way they are in sucrose, so there is no slow down at all in their absorption. This rapid metabolizing causes all kinds of health problems, he says, when HFCS is ingested in large amounts.

But is HFCS actually worse for the human body than sucrose? In a 2010 short-term study conducted at Princeton comparing uncontrolled access to fructose and sucrose, researchers showed that fructose can definitely cause problems for rats, but the results were inconsistent.[36] So the team did long-term follow-up studies, which yielded more inconsistent results. The researchers who conducted these studies feel that they have proved incontrovertibly that HFCS is bad, bad, bad. Many people agree with them. But there are also lots of objections. Some, not surprisingly, come from the corn syrup industry.[37] Some come from other, impartial, scientists who feel the method was flawed and the results contradictory.[38] What is does seem to prove, without a doubt, is that more research is needed to determine if it is just the amount of HFCS we consume which is harmful, or if it is the substance itself that causes weight gain.

Because we seem to want lots of sugar, and sugar causes problems in large amounts, wouldn't the solution, then, be to consume more artificial sweeteners? That is what the diet industry has been telling us for years. The next chapter takes a look at 'fake' sugars, and how they are processed by our bodies.

Chapter Three: Artificial Sweeteners

The nine most terrifying words in the English language are "I'm from the government, and I'm here to help."

Ronald Regan

I started drinking diet soda when I was a tween in the early 1980s. It was the thing to do. It never would have occurred to me to drink water. Soft drink makers had just replaced saccharin with aspartame based sweeteners that tasted a whole lot better, because saccharin had been found to cause bladder cancer in rats (in 2000, the FDA removed saccharin from its carcinogen list because it was found that the mechanism that caused that cancer in rats was not relevant to humans).[39] The new aspartame based sweeteners didn't have the nasty aftertaste that saccharin had. I drank two to three sodas a day. In fact, I soon preferred the taste of NutraSweet and Equal to regular sugar.

I wasn't the only one. All of my friends drank diet soda too. We drank it for years and years. For decades.

About ten years ago, though, it occurred to me that everyone I knew who drank diet soda was, well, fat. And when I looked in strangers' shopping carts, I noticed that overweight people often purchased 'diet' products. This got me thinking. Do artificial sweeteners contribute to weight gain?

And then two people I loved developed breast cancer; women, who, when tested, didn't have the breast cancer gene. They were two of the biggest diet soda consumers I knew. Did artificial sweeteners contribute to their breast cancer?

The first thing I did was to stop consuming 'fake' sugar, to the best of my ability. Because it is in so many products, it is sometimes hard to identify. Giving up diet soda was not the easiest thing I have ever done. It was the habit of a lifetime. Sometimes, I still gaze longingly at soda fountains. But it wasn't the hardest thing I've ever done, either. I replaced my diet soda consumption with water and sometimes iced tea flavored only with lemon. I get most of my caffeine through black coffee (which I love almost as much as my children).

The second thing I did was research because it is always better to light a candle than to curse the sweetness. Here is what I have found:

Types of Artificial Sweetener

At present, seven non-calorific artificial sweeteners (NAS) are approved for use in food products in the US. Think of them as horsehair wigs, instead of natural or bottled hair color. These products are so much sweeter than sucrose, manufacturers add maltodextrin (a grain starch) to the packages sold to consumers so that users can substitute equivalent amounts instead of using tweezers to pick out a few grains. Maltodextrin adds 15 calories per teaspoon, but, and I don't understand why this is, the sweeteners are still counted as zero calorie. The seven sweeteners are:

Saccharin
Brand names: Sweet n' Low®, Sugar Twin® and Necta Sweet®.

Discovered accidently in the late 1870s by a coal tar researcher who didn't wash his hands before dinner, saccharin has been commercially available since the beginning of the twentieth century.[40] Saccharin is a sodium or calcium salt that contains zero calories because your body does not digest it. It is anywhere from 200 to 700 times sweeter than sucrose. It has a strong metallic or bitter aftertaste, so companies often combine it with other sweeteners to make it taste more like sugar. It has a long shelf life, but it breaks down at higher temperatures so it isn't much good for baking.

Saccharin has been controversial since its inception, either worshipped or demonized by various segments of the population from the time of Teddy Roosevelt until now. When sugar was rationed during the first and second world wars, it became a household staple.[41] Saccharin reached its popularity zenith in the 1960s and 1970s when diet soda became a 'thing'.

In 1981, the FDA in the US required saccharin to be labeled as possibly harmful, due to the above-mentioned rat study. Interestingly, they didn't ban it because it was so popular with the public, even though they were expected to by The Delaney Amendment, which says they may not approve substances that "induce cancer in man, or, after tests, [are] found to induce cancer in animals." Then in 2000, the FDA removed the labelling requirement because it was determined not to cause cancer in people. In fact, saccharin is now often cited as among the safest artificial sweeteners out there.[42]

Aspartame
Brand names: NutraSweet®, AminoSweet® and Equal®.

Aspartame was also discovered by accident, this time in 1965, by a scientist who was trying to find an ulcer treatment, and he licked his finger while he was working.[43] It is made by combining two amino acids (protein building blocks), phenylalanine, and aspartic acid. Your body metabolizes it as aspartate, phenylalanine, and methanol. Methanol (think moonshine) turns to formaldehyde in the body, and though I want that to freak you out, many fruit juices also contain methanol. It has less than 5 calories per gram.[44] Aspartame is at least 200 sweeter than sucrose, has a comparatively short shelf life (6 months), and loses its sweetness at temperatures above 85 degrees F.

Aspartame was approved by the FDA in 1981 under a huge cloud of suspicion. Some of the controversy was because of the taint on saccharin, and some because of the sloppy trials and disingenuous analysis of the data performed by the manufacturer. [45] Aspartame is one of the most widely used NAS, and has been called 'safe' by the FDA, the American Cancer Society, and many other credible organizations, except that it is required to carry a warning for people who have phenylketonuria.

And yet, a 2007 study conducted on rats in Italy concluded that aspartame causes leukemia, lymphoma, and breast cancer, as well as other cancers.[46] The study was significant in that is used more than 4000 rats and followed them over the entire course of their natural lives.[47] The FDA contests the findings, pointing to flaws in the study and referencing other, shorter-term studies in humans that didn't show the same outcome.[48] And there *are* obvious flaws in the study, not the least of which is that the levels of aspartame used were absurdly high. The top end was 1000 times the daily limit set by the FDA, and the level where the cancer started to become pronounced was twice the FDA limit, roughly 39 cans of diet soda per day for a 165 pound person.

While I don't know anyone who consumes 39 cans of soda per day, the two women I know who developed breast cancer drank at least a two-liter bottle daily. Aspartame is in so many products from gum to yogurt, it isn't completely out of the question that someone might exceed safe limits regularly without realizing it, particularly a child, who needs to consume much less.[49] Other consumer groups, like The Center for Science in the Public Interest, urge people to avoid aspartame because of this and different trials that show it is harmful to fetuses.

Other studies have linked aspartame to a number of different health conditions including headaches, dizziness, kidney failure, and strokes, though it has not been proved beyond a shadow of a doubt that aspartame causes these conditions.[50] The majority of FDA complaints each year are about aspartame.[51]

Pepsi recently announced they are pulling aspartame from their products, though whether it is because they think it is harmful or they are just sick of public outcry is unclear.[52]

Acesulfame potassium (also called acesulfame K and Ace K)
Brand names: Sunett® and Sweet One®

Ace K is produced by combining acetoacetic acid with potassium. Acetoacetic acid, according to the Miller-Keane

Encyclopedia and Dictionary of Medicine is, "one of the ketone bodies formed in the body in the metabolism of certain substances, particularly in the liver in the combustion of fats. It is present in the body in increased amounts in abnormal conditions such as uncontrolled diabetes mellitus and starvation."[53] It is not absorbed in the body except for a bit of potassium.

Ace K was discovered in 1967, in the usual way, by accident, by a chemist who licked his fingers to pick up a piece of paper. I was unable to find what he was working on at the time, but in the late 1960s the company he was working for, Horst AG, was a leader in diuretics and diabetic medication.[54] Ace K is 200 times sweeter than sugar. It was first approved by the FDA in 1992.[55] It has a 3-4 year shelf life and is stable at high temperatures.

Ace K is often mixed with other NAS, especially aspartame to cancel out the bitter taste.[56] It is also often used to sweeten tart drinks, like lemonade.[57] It has been found to stimulate insulin release.

The Center for Science in the Public Interest has Ace K on their no-fly list because the safety studies conducted in the 1970s were sketchy. In newer studies, it has been linked to cancer and thyroid problems in animals, but not in people.[58]

Sucralose
Brand name: Splenda®

As the name suggests, sucralose is modified sucrose. Three hydrogen-oxygen groups in the sugar are replaced with chlorine ions and the resulting crystal is 600 times sweeter than sucrose. It lasts longer and is more heat tolerant than saccharin and aspartame. In fact, the crystals don't melt when you bake them like sugar does. People metabolize about 15% of sucralose, and the rest passes through the body. It was discovered in 1976, wait for it, by accident, by a foreign graduate student who was helping to research industrial applications of modified sucrose at a British sugar company. He misheard the command 'test it' as 'taste it.'[59] Bodabing!

After intensive testing, the FDA approved sucralose in 1998. It is considered 'safe' by the FDA and the health watchdog organizations of many other countries. Pepsi recently announced they were switching from aspartame to sucralose for its diet products.

When it was first commercially available, Splenda used the tagline, "Made from sugar, so it tastes like sugar." They wanted to give off the image that it was only slightly processed to remove the calories, call to mind products like decaf coffee and non-fat milk. Just spin it around in a centrifuge and the calories come right out! This is tantamount to saying, "Hydrogen peroxide: Water, now with extra oxygen!" Competitors and watchdogs have forced Splenda to tack on the phrase "But it's not sugar" to its tagline.

Neotame
Brand name: NewTame®

Neotame is a derivative of aspartame, but much, much sweeter. It is 7000 to 13000 times sweeter than sucrose. Unusually for a synthetic sweetener, neotame was developed on purpose by Monsansto, the makers of NutraSweet. It was approved by the FDA in 2002.[60]

Neotame breaks down into two substances in the body, and the only one the body metabolizes is methanol (but much less than aspartame).[61] You won't find packages of neotame in the coffee cart because it is mainly sold to manufacturers. It has a couple of advantages over other NAS. Because so much less is required, it is by far the cheapest sweetener for manufacturers to use. Also, it holds up to temperature better than aspartame so it can be used in baked goods.

Although it has been tainted by its connection to aspartame, the watchdog group The Center for Science in the Public Interest declares it to be one of the very few safe sweeteners out there.[62] Of course, there are dissenters. Dr. Joseph Mercola points out that it is used in cattle fodder because it increases the cows' appetites.[63]

Advantame

Advantame is Japanese aspartame with some vanillin thrown in. It is sweeter than aspartame, by several orders of magnitude. In fact, it is 20,000 times sweeter than sugar.[64] It was developed on purpose and was approved by the FDA in 2014. Because it is so much sweeter than aspartame and so much less is required, it does not come with the warning for people who have phenylketonuria. Even the Center for Science in the Public Interest seems to feel it is safe because the amount consumed is darn near negligible.

Stevia

Brand names: Truvia®, PureVia®

Stevia comes from the *Stevia rebaudiana* (Bertoni) plant native to South America. Indigenous people there have used the leaves as a sweetener and medicine for centuries. But it only 'kind of' comes from the plant, because the FDA has not approved the whole leaf or "crude' extracts from the plant because of concerns regarding, "control of blood sugar and effects on the reproductive, cardiovascular, and renal systems."[65]

What was approved for general use by the FDA in 2008 is a highly processed extract known as Rebaudioside A (or Reb A). This extract is 200 times sweeter than sugar. Companies like Coca-Cola, which makes Truvia, use dozens of processes and chemicals like acetone, and methanol to extract the sweetness.[66]

Catherine Ulbricht, senior pharmacist at Massachusetts General Hospital, says that stevia may help with hypertension and that it lowers blood sugar levels. It also may interact with a variety of prescriptions like antifungals, anti-inflammatories, antimicrobials, anti-cancer drugs, cholesterol-lowering agents, fertility drugs, and a host of other medications, so she cautions people to talk to their doctor before consuming it.[67]

The Center for Science in the Public Interest lists stevia as safe but warns that they do not feel it has been adequately tested for cancer. They say that "several (but not all) genetic tests found that rebiana-related substances caused mutations and other forms of genotoxicity."[68]

General health concerns

None of these substances has thus far been proven to the FDA to cause harm to consumers who use them in reasonable amounts. But just because something has so far not been proven to cause cancer it doesn't follow that the substance is either safe or good for you. And I would argue, most fervently, that it isn't the government's job to police what is on your dinner place. If they know a substance is dangerous, then by all means that data should be made public. But it is unreasonable to expect that the government should understand the far-reaching health consequences of every substance that we come into contact with. And even if it *was* their job, political agencies have a divided agenda where facts compete with economic consideration and popular opinion. As individuals, we have much more accountability for what we put into our bodies; therefore, we have more responsibility understand them. This extends far beyond artificial sweeteners.

Raises blood sugar level higher than sucrose?

Conventional wisdom says that using artificial sweeteners has no effect on blood sugar levels. Why would they? They don't introduce sugar into the blood. But in 2014, a team of researchers at the Weizmann Institute of Science in Israel discovered that saccharin, aspartame, and sucralose all alter gut bacteria in a way that, in some mice and people, makes them glucose intolerant (hyperglycemic).[69]

The researchers added a 10% solution of either saccharin, aspartame, sucralose, or glucose to the drinking water of mice (there was a water only control group), and gave some a regular diet, and some a high-fat diet. The amount of sweetener they consumed was the equivalent of four mice-sized cans of cola. After 11 weeks the scientists reported that the blood sugar levels of some of each group of the artificial sweetener fed mice were *higher* than the sugar-fed mice, regardless of whether they had a regular or high-fat diet. They were "almost diabetic".[70]

"Initially, we were surprised by the results, which is why we also repeated them multiple times," said Eran Segal, Ph.D., one of the leads in the project.

Next the researchers gave the mice with the high blood sugar levels antibiotics for four weeks, and their blood sugar dropped back to normal. Then, the scientists implanted the feces of untreated high blood sugar mice into mice with normal blood sugar levels, and the mice who received the poop transplant saw a spike in their blood sugar.[71]

Do artificial sweeteners cause the same blood sugar spikes in people? The researchers looked at the gut bacteria of 400 people, and found that on average, those who regularly consumed artificial sweeteners had higher fasting blood sugar levels than those who didn't, and they also had a higher frequency of glucose intolerance. So they recruited a pool of 7 healthy people who didn't consume artificial sweeteners and performed a variation of the mouse experiment on them. They fed the people the maximum acceptable limit of saccharin per day (as determined by the FDA) for a week. After seven days, four of the people high blood sugar levels. When the researchers implanted the feces from those four people into mice, the blood sugar in the mice elevated.

Critics of the study say that the human sample size was too small, that the researchers combined the data from all three NAS and that it might relate only to saccharin, and that hysteria over the results might lead people to believe that consuming sugar is a healthier choice than artificial sweeteners.[72] What everyone seems to agree on, however, is that that more research is warranted.

Causes more weight gain than sugar?

Many people use NAS to avoid weight gain, but study after study has shown that artificial sweeteners cause more weight gain than sugar.

For example, a 2013 study in Brazil looked at NAS intake and weight gain among rats. Along with unlimited rat chow, some were fed yogurt sweetened with aspartame, some yogurt sweetened with saccharin, and some yogurt sweetened with sucrose. All consumed a similar number of calories, which means that the rats eating NAS felt driven to eat more rat chow that the rats who ate the yogurt sweetened with sugar.

Despite the similar caloric intake, both the saccharin and aspartame groups gained more weight than the sugar group.[73] The researchers were unsure why these results were achieved, and speculated that, even though activity was restricted for all rats, the sugar-fed rats somehow expended more energy and retained less water than the NAS fed rats.[74]

One Yale researcher looked at all of the different studies where the subjects gained more weight eating NAS than sucrose or glucose, and explained the results this way: sweet tastes increase appetite. The natural sweeteners glucose and fructose provide energy which somehow triggers a response in the body that says 'enough.' They activate the food reward area of the brain. NAS do not. The artificial sugars just make you hungrier.[75] In other words, artificial sugars compel people to eat.

There are more studies and more analysis of artificial sweeteners and weight gain. Some say that aspartame raises insulin and leptin (a hormone that regulates fat storage) and over time cause your body to become less sensitive to both, driving weight gain and diabetes.[76] Some say that NAS lowers your metabolism.[77] But what they all point to, is that there is no free lunch, no way of eating your cake and having it too, no way to indiscriminately add sweet food to your diet without health consequences.

'Diet' sugars are not a healthy alternative to 'natural' and 'processed' sugars. When regulating your sugar intake, it is paramount that you eliminate artificial sweeteners.

Chapter Four: How Does Too Much Sugar Prevent Weight Loss?

"I want to lose weight by eating nothing but moon pies, which have significantly less gravity than earthier foods such as fruits and vegetables."
— *Jarod Kintz*

Weight gain and loss should be a simple math exercise, like the greater than/less than alligator signs from elementary school. If you eat more calories than you burn, you will store those calories as fat and gain weight. If you burn more calories than you consume, you will burn body fat. But an excess of sugar screws up the natural fat regulation process in several different ways.

The first is that when you consume a lot of sugar, your body begins to absorb a higher percentage of the sugar that you eat. One study found that obese children absorbed 100% of the fructose they ate and drank into their livers, whereas lean kids absorbed only about half of the sugar and eliminated the rest.[78] Their bodies metabolized the sugar differently. Dr. Richard Johnson, head of nephrology at The University of Colorado, says that this is because the more fructose a person ingests, the more the receptors in their digestive tracts get 'turned on' and allow it to pass to the liver, versus eliminating it as waste. So it turns out that sugary and high starch foods really are more fattening for overweight people than for lean folks.

Another reason that sugar causes weight gain is that both insulin resistance and chronic fructose consumption can trigger a resistance to a hormone called leptin, which regulates long-term fat storage.[79],[80] Leptin is produced by your fat cells. The more body fat you have, the more leptin your cells produce. Your brain monitors the leptin level in your blood and recognizes when there is enough. When the levels are sufficient, your brain tells you that you are full, and tells your body to begin burning fat. When it senses that leptin levels are low, it tells you that you are starving and that you should eat. It also tells you to stop burning fat and to stop expending energy so you don't die. [81] It is an efficient regulator. The problem is that lots of fructose, insulin resistance, high triglycerides, and inflammation can interfere with the brain's ability to correctly read leptin levels. It stops sending 'full' signals, and people begin to overeat. In fact, even though there is an abundance of leptin in the bloodstream, because the brain no longer recognizes it, it tells the body that *it is starving*, even when calorie consumption is sufficient, or in excess. The brain tells the body to keep eating and to stop burning fat!

One of the keys to increasing your sensitivity to leptin is to dramatically reduce sugar and starch. Dr. Jeremy E. Kaslow says that even an occasional sugary treat can disrupt your fat burning for 2-3 days![82] While this doesn't mean you can't ever enjoy another brownie again, it does mean that you have to reset the way your body works first, so that when you do indulge, you will be satisfied with it, and not immediately feel an intense craving for more.

Increasing fiber can also help increase your sensitivity to leptin. Fiber can help decrease gut inflammation, one of the triggers that cause the body to ignore leptin.

But just fixing your sensitivity to leptin doesn't solve all of your weight loss problems. Not right away. Leptin is also the reason that when you begin a new diet and start losing weight, your body begins to sabotage you. When you lose fat, your now properly leptin sensitive body notices that there is a decrease in leptin being produced by your fat cells, and it determines that you are starving. Your energy level drops and you find yourself hungrier than ever because your brain is trying to keep you from dying. It doesn't recognize that you have too much fat, only that your fat reserves are depleting, and the survival mechanisms kick in. To combat your hormones while you lose weight, it is critical to eat lots of fiber, protein, and good fat, and to eat enough calories regularly to prevent starvation mode from kicking in.[83]

The next chapter covers the specifics for managing sugar cravings and keeping your hunger hormones under control while you go through your sugar detox.

Chapter Five: 10-Day Sugar Detox Guidelines

*"It is our choices, Harry, that show what we truly are,
far more than our abilities."*
— *J. K. Rowling*

My husband operates on the theory that if he makes at least 51% good choices, be it in life, finances, diet, or child rearing, then the equation will balance out in his favor. The trouble with this line of reasoning is that you have to keep careful track to know whether you are in the red or the black.

And, unfortunately, that kind of obsessive attention is required, at least at first, when you are weaning your body off of sugar.

Discerning your Sugar Intake

We said earlier that experts recommend 6 teaspoons or less of added sugar for women per day. But packages don't list sugar in teaspoons, they list it in grams. One teaspoon of sugar is 4 grams, so women need to keep their added sugar consumption under 24 grams, and men need to keep theirs below 36 grams.

We also said that complex carbohydrates break down into sugar and that carbs ought to be limited as well. For people who are active, at a healthy body weight, and are not diabetic or pre-diabetic, 100 to 150 grams of carbs per day is a healthy goal. For those trying to lose weight, try to keep carbs below 100 grams.

BUT - In order to give your body a chance to get over a sugar addiction, it is necessary to strictly limit the more complex sugar as well as the easily accessible stuff for the first 10 days. During the 10-Day sugar detox, you should avoid all added sugars and artificial sweeteners, and severely limit grains, milk products, and sweet fruit. Most of the things that come in a package or with a label are going to be off limits.

That is a lot of restrictions. And you will miss the sugar. At first. But as you go through the ten days, your body will begin to release less insulin. This will have a number of effects. Your body will release the excess water it has been hoarding causing that incredible initial, but sadly unsustainable, weight drop that happens at the beginning of low carb diets. What is sustainable, though is that you will stop storing fat and start burning fat, which your body will not do when your insulin levels are high and causing problems with your leptin sensitivity.[84] And after several days, you will stop craving the sugar.

To counteract the lack of sugar, you will need to increase protein and fat. Yep, fat. But, unfortunately, we're not talking unlimited bacon here. That fat you will need more of is healthy fat, found in foods like olive oil, avocados, nuts, and legumes. Once your body realizes that it can use this fat as fuel, you will be sated and full of energy.

How to count carbs

One of the problems of eliminating packaged food, at least for the first ten days, is that it is hard to count the calories, grams of protein, carbs, fiber, etc. in foods that don't come with a label. And if you are eating leans meats, vegetables, nuts, seeds, eggs, and legumes, you shouldn't need to. But if you'd like to, one of the ways you can do it is by using an online calculator. I like the one at caloriecount.com because you can enter a recipe and the number of servings, and it will spit out all the data. That is the calculator I used for the recipes in this book. You can plan a week's worth of meals if you like, and get your food plan for the duration in order.

Once you know the approximate number of carbs in a meal, subtract the fiber, because your body doesn't break that down. Aim to get less than half of your calories from carbs while on the 10-Day sugar detox. The other half should come from protein and fat.

Beverages to avoid

Beverages are an especially sneaky place for sugar to hide. During the first ten days, it is critical to watch the beverages you consume. In fact, I'd say to limit your drinks to black coffee, black, green, and herbal tea, and water.

Alcohol is out for two reasons. The first is that it contains sugar. The second is that it lowers your willpower and tempts you into eating an entire carton of ice cream. After ten days, you can add a drink or two back into your day per your doctor's recommendations. The traditional guideline is up to one drink a day for women, and up to two for men.

Cream and sweeteners, including and especially artificial ones, are a no-no for coffee. This includes milk substitutes like soy and rice. Once you make it the ten days, you can add them back if you desire, if that is how you want to spend your daily sugar allotment. Also, watch out for sugar content in flavored coffees.

Sodas and juices are prohibited, whether they are regular or diet because either will increase your sugar cravings. The only exception would be juices you make yourself, out of vegetables, such as a homemade green smoothies with a water base.

Avoid dairy during the ten-day sugar detox, again for two reasons. The first is that dairy contains sugar. The second is that many people have a lactose sensitivity they are unaware of that makes them crave dairy, even though it causes inflammation.[85] The gut inflammation messes with their insulin and leptin sensitivities. Bizarre, but true.

Foods to avoid

Unfortunately, it is probably easier to list foods that are on the table versus those that are off. If you stick to lean meats, fish, vegetables, nuts, seeds, and legumes, you will do great. But here is a breakdown of the major categories of foods to avoid:

Packaged foods – because during processing nutrients are stripped out and sugar and salt are added.

Dairy – as described in the beverages to avoid section, dairy contains sugar and many people have undiagnosed dairy sensitivities. You can add dairy back in after the ten days.

Trans fat – Trans fats are formerly healthy fats that have been hydrogenated to stay solid at room temperature and not spoil. Trans fats drastically increase all sorts of bad processes in the body, including heart disease, diabetes, and inflammation. "There is no safe level of consumption," according to the Institute of Medicine.[86]

High fructose fruits – Avoid the fruits that are highest in fructose, such as watermelon, cherries, mangoes, apples, and pears. Also avoid dried fruits.

Foods to increase

Protein, protein, and protein! When you limit your intake of carbohydrates and sugars, then your body must search for an alternative source of energy. Fat stored in the body cannot be converted into glucose; protein can. Protein has been found in many studies to increase your feeling of fullness after meals, and it will also stimulate the release of insulin.

You should get 20-30% of your calories from lean, healthy protein.

Unsaturated fats - Depending on which source you trust, somewhere between 20-35% of your calories should come from healthy fats. Fish, lean meats, poultry, nuts, seeds, and olive oil are great sources of good fat.

Making it easier on yourself

Detoxing from sugar is going to require some willpower, no two ways about it. But there are a number of things you can do before and during the detox to set yourself up for success.

Exercise

Exercise promotes insulin sensitivity, according to diabetes researcher Joseph Henson, Ph.D. from the University of Leicester. He says that it helps both healthy people and people with type 2 diabetes. And it isn't just exercise, it is the art of not being sedentary for too long. So while a workout at the gym is fantastic, if that isn't already a part of your routine, start by thinking smaller. Aim to take a break from sitting every hour. Set an alarm and walk around the office. Refill your water glass. "We found that it was the amount of time that people spent sitting that had the biggest impact on glucose, triglycerides, and HDL cholesterol and not the level of exercise," he said. "This just shows what a negative impact too much sitting can have on an individual's health, independent of the level of exercise."[87]

Stand up while you work, take the stairs, do everything you can to keep from sitting too much throughout the day.

Plan ahead of time how you are going to get your exercise each day, and stick to the exercise plan the same way you are going to stick to your eating routine.

Get Enough Sleep

Getting enough sleep is just as critical as exercise in fighting your sugar addiction. This is because when you don't get enough sleep, you are more likely to overeat, crave sugary foods, and not exercise.[88] Study after study has shown that when you don't get enough sleep, you crave high carb foods and you lack impulse control. By getting at least eight hours of sleep a night, you are going to make the 10-Day sugar detox infinitely easier on yourself.

Clean Your Cupboards

Before starting the 10-Day Sugar Detox, remove temptation. Remove sugary and packaged food from your house. I would go as far as removing bread, pasta, rice, and baking supplies. If you want to permanently get rid of them, take them to a homeless shelter. If not, store them in an airtight container and put them in a friend's garage for two weeks. If the temptation isn't easily accessible, it won't call to you during your weakest moments.

Shop and prep ahead of time

Once you clean out the junk food from your shelves, fill them with the healthy foods you will eat for your detox. Plan out your meals and snacks ahead of time, and shop and prep for them as much as you can before you begin your detox. Make some of the dishes and condiments in advance, like the breakfast egg cups, nut butter, homemade salad dressing, sugar-free ketchup, Chimmichuri Sauce, etc. Not having to decide what to eat on an empty stomach, or shop when you are hangry, can make all the difference between success and failure.

Clear Your Calendar

Schedule your sugar detox during a lower stress time. Don't do it when you are travelling, around the holidays, during an important project at work, or any other time when you have more than normal going on. Many women experience additional cravings before and during their periods, so that may not be an optimal time. Plan to eat in every night during the detox. If you are going to get together with friends or family, be the host so you can control the menu.

Eat Regularly

Plan three meals and two snacks each day ahead of time, and eat them on schedule. It is harder to resist cravings when you are hungry.

Plan for Cravings

What can you do when temptation strikes? Plan how you are going to handle it ahead of time. Keep trainers on hand so you can go for a walk around the block. Have healthy snacks nearby so you can eat a hand full of nuts or blackberries. One of my favorite treats is Kind® bars, which provide lots of protein, and only 4 grams of sugar. Keep some Ibuprofen in your desk drawer in case a headache hits you. Having strategies mapped out will make you feel more powerful during a vulnerable time. And don't wait for the cravings to get intense to put your intervention into action. Act at the first sign and dominate them.

Keep in mind that not all sugar cravings are physical. Many are emotional. People use sugar as both a reward and as a pacifier. We turn to it when we are upset and angry, when we are depressed, when we are stressed, when we want to celebrate, when we are bored. Have a strategy in place to recognize and combat emotional cravings. Arm yourself with as many weapons as you can.

> Call a good friend who makes you feel loved or makes you laugh.

> Read a short excerpt from a funny writer (my favorites are Dave Barry and David Sedaris). I keep a paperback copy of a book in my purse and read an essay when I need to laugh. Follow funny bloggers.

> Have music on your mp3 player that makes you feel good. Download Pandora on your computer and have music that you have positive associations with quietly in the background.

> Post pictures around you that make you happy be it of loved ones, yourself in a bikini, cats playing, or famous paintings. Try to keep your surrounding free of clutter so that your visual environment does not stress you out.

> Use essential oils or scented candles to surround yourself with scents that have positive associations for you. Before you go to work, dab some cinnamon or

lemon oil on a cotton ball and keep it in a plastic bag. Pull it out when you need a pick me up.

Seal your Meals with Fruit

A fruit at the end of a long day or after lunch will help put a "seal" on your sugar intake for that particular portion of the day. The sugar in the fruit should trick your brain into believing that it has gotten its necessary reward, and your brain should respond by no longer craving sugar, even if it is just for a couple of hours.

Many health professionals agree that having at least one serving of fruit with every meal is advisable. This one serving helps to spike sugar levels in the blood, though more gradually than with processed sugars because of the fiber. Choose fruits that are lower in fructose, such as berries, kiwis, bananas, and oranges.

These fruits should provide a steady flow of sugar into the bloodstream, and just like with the "slow" carbohydrates, this should help curb the side effects of sugar detox. Symptoms such as cravings, anxiety, insomnia, mood swings, and irritability, if they are a problem, should decrease in their severity as your body starts to truly adjust to living with less sugar, usually by the fourth day. After the fourth day, begin to reduce the amount of fruit you are eating to 1 ½ - 2 servings daily.

What happens if you cheat?

If you happen to fall off the sugar wagon, don't despair. Do stop and take note of how your feel. Did the treat satisfy your sugar craving, or did it leave you wanting more? Realizing the effects of sugar can be useful in keeping yourself motivated to stay with your plan in the future. After that, forgive yourself and move on. All is not lost, and all your hard work has not been spoiled. Tomorrow is another day.

Chapter Six: The Ten Day Sugar Detox

Setting a goal is not the main thing. It is deciding how you will go about achieving it and staying with that plan.

Tom Landry

This is a very general plan for detoxing from sugar over a ten-day period. The meal plan and recipes offered are just suggestions. All of the dishes are tasty and kid-friendly in my house, but feel free to substitute with your own favorites and new experiments as you like. Note that the fruit serving sizes decrease after the first four days so that you are consuming a maximum of two fruit servings per day.

Make sure you drink plenty of water. Other acceptable beverages are black coffee, unsweetened iced tea, unsweetened black tea, and unsweetened herbal tea.

Day One:

You've shopped, you've prepped, and you got a good night's sleep. Your walking shoes are already in the car for a quick stroll after work. Your determination and sense of purpose are high. Let's do this!

As you eat throughout the day, try to savor every bite. Enjoy your mealtime; take a break from work and electronic devices.

If you are tempted by sugary treats, remind yourself that you are fighting a physical addiction and that rather than satisfying your craving, giving in is likely to increase it.

Alter your typical routine today, especially during times when you traditionally indulge in desserts or high-carb treats. Take a walk after dinner. Fold laundry or polish old shoes while you are watching TV. Keep your hands busy.

Suggested Meals:

Breakfast: 2 Turkey Sausage Egg Cups (p. 59) , 1 small banana

Mid-morning snack: 1 oz. nuts

Lunch: Turkey Wraps (p. 71) , 1 cup of strawberries

Afternoon snack: 1 oz. Nut Butter (p. 110) and celery sticks

Dinner: Baked Salmon (p. 82) and Sautéed Spinach with Salsa (p. 98) , 1 Orange

Day Two:

Hopefully, you still feel great and motivated today. You slept well, and you're ready to knock out another day.

Throughout the day, you might start to feel a more intense sugar craving. This could include irritability, headaches, fatigue, depression, anxiety, and shakiness, in addition to feeling drawn to sugar, bread, chips, etc. You may have trouble sleeping tonight.

Keep your coping mechanisms close at hand. Have healthy

snack food ready, and move about frequently throughout the day. Try to enjoy your meals, savoring the sweet fruit. Vary your routine, especially during times when you would normally snack on desserts or chips, etc.

Suggested Meals:

Breakfast: Eggs Your Way (p. 65) , 1 cup of cantaloupe

Mid-morning snack: 1 oz. roasted pumpkin seeds

Lunch: Spicy Tuna Rolls (p. 73), 1 orange

Afternoon snack: Fresh and Sweet "Orange" Juice (p. 102)

Dinner: Lemon Basil Chicken (p. 75), Roasted Brussel Sprouts (p. 92), 1 peach

Day Three:

Today and tomorrow are going to be the hardest. You might be cranky and tired throughout the day. Fight it with added exercise, a walk after lunch or dinner, taking the stairs when you can, an extra lap around the parking lot.

Take time to enjoy your meals. Feel the energy from your food course through your body. Visualize it travelling through bloodstream to your muscles. Enjoy the sweetness from the fruit. Remember when you are tempted by carbs and sweets that your body is fighting hard to overcome an addiction. You will probably be tempted a lot today. Use all of your coping strategies to get past the temptations.

Reward yourself with a hot bath and a good book after

dinner, or another relaxing activity you enjoy. Take time for yourself today.

Suggested Meals:
Breakfast: Antioxidant Kale Green Smoothie (p. 61)

Mid-morning snack: 1 Turkey Sausage Egg Cup (p. 59)

Lunch: Pesto Egg Salad Wraps (p. 69), 2 kiwi fruit

Afternoon snack: ¼ Cup Hummus (p. 104) and cut up vegetables

Dinner: Roast Pork Tenderloin (p. 84), Boiled Green Beans with Lemon (p. 96), 1 plum

Day Four:

After today, any cravings you have should start to abate. Continue using your coping skills to resist sweets and high-carb foods. If your sleep has been rough, limit screen time before bed and give yourself plenty of time to unwind. If you don't already stretch each day, consider adding in some easy stretching to your morning and evening routines.

Keep up your daily exercise. Make some time for yourself as well. Do something today that feeds your soul.

Suggested Meals:
Breakfast: 2 Turkey Sausage Egg Cups (p 59.), ½ grapefruit

Mid-morning snack: 1 oz. roasted sunflower seeds

Lunch: Leftover Salad (p. 67)

Afternoon snack: 1 cup sugar snap peas

Dinner: Pork 'Tacos' (p. 86) , 1 cup mango or papaya

Day Five:

Today you should start to feel more energized. Saying 'no' when people offer your treats shouldn't be as hard.

Your body should be able to tolerate less sugar. Begin to cut back on the amount of fruit you consume, cutting down the portions to 1 ½-2 servings per day, the recommended guidelines for adults.

Suggested Meals:
Breakfast: Caprese Egg Cups (p. 63), ½ cup blackberries

Mid-morning snack: Fresh and Sweet "Orange" Juice (p. 102)

Lunch: Turkey Wraps (p. 71) , ½ orange

Afternoon snack: ¼ cup Hummus (p. 104) and cut up vegetables

Dinner: Leftovers, ½ cup of strawberries

By now you should be getting used to filling up at each meal on vegetables, healthy proteins, and healthy fats. Take some time today to seek out new recipes and foods that will make eating a reduced sugar diet in the future easier. Think about trying fruits and vegetables that you have previously shunned in the past or have never tried before. Remember, it can take your palate up to twenty experiences with a food before you really know if you like it or not.

Suggested Meals:

Breakfast: Eggs Your Way (p. 65) , ½ banana

Mid-morning snack: 1 oz. roasted almonds

Lunch: Spicy Tuna Rolls (p. 73), 1 plum

Afternoon snack: ¼ cup Guacamole (p. 106) with cut up vegetables

Dinner: Steamed edamame followed by Catfish Soup (p. 80), ½ cup raspberries

Day Seven:

Continue to focus on increasing your daily activity and sleeping enough each night.

As you experience any cravings today for sugary or high-carb foods, try to notice the particulars of the situation. Do they happen when you are hungry? When you are happy or under a lot of stress? Do sugary or high-carb foods act as a reward or a tonic for you? Be an observer of your triggers.

Also spend time today thinking away ways to reward yourself that don't involve food. Think about experiences you enjoy and how you can replace food rewards with behaioral ones.

Suggested Meals:
Breakfast: Antioxidant Kale Green Smoothie (p. 61)

Mid-morning snack: 2 tbsp. Nut Butter (p.110) with celery

Lunch: Pesto Egg Salad Wraps (p. 69) , ½ Orange

Afternoon snack: 1 cup sugar snap peas

Dinner: Almond Chicken Fingers (p. 78) with Steamed Cauliflower (p. 94), 1 kiwi fruit

Day Eight:

Focus today on the energy that you have. Pay attention to how you feel before and after you exercise. Observe your energy levels before and after you eat.

Spend time today thinking about activities that you enjoy now or would like to incorporate into your life to a greater extent in the future. Take a look at all of the 'how-to' videos available on YouTube, everything from yoga to skiing. Check out the classes that are available at your local rec center or gym.

Breakfast: Caprese Egg Cups (p. 63), ½ cup cantaloupe

Mid-morning snack: 1 oz. roasted pumpkin seeds

Lunch: Leftover Salad (p. 67)

Afternoon snack: ¼ cup Guacamole (p. 106) with cut up vegetables

Dinner: Buffaloaf (p. 88) with Roasted Asparagus (p. 92), 1 apricot

Day Nine:

Start thinking today about a long-term eating strategy. What about the last nine days has been hard? What have you enjoyed? What strategies have you learned that will help you continue to eat a reduced sugar diet as you carry forward?

What are your long-term health and fitness goal? Take time today to write down what you would like to accomplish and by when. Then write down ideas about how you will get there. Are there medications you would like to discontinue? Weight you would like to drop? Activities you would like to be able to participate in, but you do not yet have the vitality to do so? Use the success you have had over the last nine days as a springboard for future success.

Suggested Meals:
Breakfast: Eggs Your Way (p. 65), ½ grapefruit

Mid-morning snack: 2 tbsp. Nut Butter (p. 110) with celery

Lunch: Turkey Wraps (p. 71), 1 orange

Afternoon snack: ¼ cup Hummus (p. 104) with cut up vegetables

Dinner: Leftovers, ½ peach

Day Ten:

Focus today on gratitude. Congratulate yourself for completing the Ten Day Sugar Detox. Appreciate today the things in your life that make you happy.

Suggested Meals:
Breakfast: Antioxidant Kale Green Smoothie (p. 61)

Mid-morning snack: 2 tbsp. Nut Butter (p. 110) with celery

Lunch: Pesto Egg Salad Wraps (p. 69), ½ cup berries

Afternoon snack: ¼ cup Guacamole (p. 106) with cut up vegetables

Dinner: Chimichurri Chicken Kabobs (p. 90) with Zoodles (p. 100) , ½ Orange

Day Eleven:

While it may be tempting to celebrate completing the Ten Day Sugar Detox by indulging in all the foods you've been missing, it is a good idea to take it slowly.

Add foods back one at a time, and observe your body's reaction to it. If you eat a cookie and immediately and intensely crave more, then your detox is not over. Continue to abstain from sugar and reduce your fruit intake for another week. If, instead, you find that you can enjoy a treat and feel satisfied, your detox was successful. Your task now is to keep your body from going back to the way it was before.

Continue to watch your added sugars and keep them to a minimum. Enjoy the sugars and simple carbs that you do consume. If weight loss is a goal, your body should be primed and ready. Keep eating a high protein/low sugar diet while exercising, and watch the weight melt away.

Be careful about consuming alcohol. Limit your intake to a glass or two per day, per your doctor's guidelines. Nothing ruins a healthy eating plan like too much alcohol.

Observe how your body reacts to dairy if you add it back into your diet. You might have noticed that your skin improved and your gut functioned better without it. If so, consider continuing to limit it in the future.

Keep looking for new healthy recipes and foods that you will want to try. The best eating plans are ones that are both healthy and tasty too, that don't leave you feeling deprived. Keep up your habit of eating fruit as a dessert. Feel free to add back in higher fructose fruits, like apples, pears, and grapes. Eat processed food as a treat, not a staple.

Chapter Seven: Recipes

Breakfast

Turkey Sausage Egg Cups

Serving Size: 2 Egg Cups, Serves 6
Prep time: 10 Min
Cook Time: 45 Min
Total Time: 1 hour

These are a great make ahead, grab and go hot breakfast that will fill you up and load you with energy. Play around with the recipe and add other veggies and spices. Eggs have a high amount of cholesterol but have been shown in many studies to increase your HDL (good cholesterol) while leaving the LDL unchanged.[89] If you are worried about it, though, feel free to use just the egg whites, or substitute Egg Beaters.

Ingredients:
- 12 Omega-3 enriched eggs
- 1 lb. ground turkey sausage
- 1 head of broccoli (or 1 package frozen broccoli)
- Olive oil cooking spray or olive oil

Instructions:
1. Preheat oven to 350 F.
2. Grease a muffin tin with olive oil cooking spray (or olive oil).
3. Boil or steam the broccoli, or prepare your favorite way.
4. Brown the ground turkey.

5. While the turkey is browning, crack the eggs into a large bowl and whisk until well mixed. Add the sausage and broccoli, and mix thoroughly. Divide the mixture evenly among the 12 muffin cups. Bake at 350 for 30 minutes. Allow to cool, and dig in.
6. You can prepare these ahead of time, store in the fridge, and reheat for 30-60 seconds in the microwave.

Nutrition Facts	
Serving Size 2 Cups	
% Based on 2000 Calorie Diet	
Per Serving	% Daily Value
Calories 267	13.35%
Calories from Fat 155	
Total Fat 17.2g	26%
Saturated Fat 4.9g	24%
Cholesterol 418mg	139%
Sodium 614mg	26%
Potassium 230mg	7%
Carbohydrates 2.8g	1%
Dietary Fiber 0.8g	3%
Sugars 1.3g	
Protein 25.6g	
Vitamin A 14%	Vitamin C 45%
Calcium 8%	Iron 11%

Antioxidant Kale Green Smoothie

Servings: 1

Total time: 5 minutes

I love green smoothies for breakfast. I buy big bags of prewashed spinach and kale, and bags of frozen fruit for quick, easy breakfasts. Substitute spinach for the kale if you prefer.

Ingredients:

- 2 c water
- 2 tbsp. almond butter (p. 110) or 1 oz. almonds
- 1 banana frozen in chunks
- 1 c frozen or fresh blueberries
- 2 tbsp. orange zest
- 2 tbsp. orange juice
- 2 c kale

Instructions:

1. Add the liquid base in the blender first.
2. Add the almond butter or almonds.
3. Add the banana.
4. Add the blueberries, orange zest, and orange juice.
5. Add the baby kale.
6. Blend at the highest speed for 30-45 seconds.

Nutrition Facts	
Serving Size 1 Serving	
% Based on 2000 Calorie Diet	
Per Serving	% Daily Value

Calories 483	24.15%
Calories from Fat 19	
Total Fat 1.8g	9%
Saturated Fat .2g	
Cholesterol 0mg	0%
Sodium 75mg	3%
Potassium 1527mg	44%
Carbohydrates 73.8g	25%
Dietary Fiber 11.1g	44%
Sugars 314g	
Protein 13.5g	
Vitamin A 415%	Vitamin C 394%
Calcium 31%	Iron 34%

Caprese Egg Cups

Serving Size – 2 egg cups
Serves: 6
Prep time: 10 min
Cook time: 30 min
Total time: 40 min

This recipe is similar to the egg cup recipe above in that you can make ahead of time, and grab and go. Reheating these tasty treats is a little harder, however, because the egg yolks will explode in the microwave. Reheat in the microwave in 10-second intervals. For best results, warm them in a skillet with a little olive oil.

Ingredients:
- 12 slices Canadian Bacon
- 12 Omega-3 enriched eggs
- 3 Roma tomatoes, cut into 4 slices each
- Fresh basil leaves washed
- Olive oil cooking spray (or olive oil)
- ¼ cup balsamic vinegar

Instructions:
1. Preheat oven to 350 F. Grease a muffin tin with olive oil spray (or olive oil). Place one slice of Canadian bacon in each muffin cup. Top with a slice of tomato and 3-4 basil leaves. Crack an egg on top. Try not to break the yolk, but it isn't a big deal if you do.
2. Bake at 350 for 30 minutes, or until the eggs are properly cooked.

3. In the meantime, simmer the vinegar until reduced by half.
4. Drizzle the eggs with the vinegar reduction.

Nutrition Facts	
Serving Size 1 Serving	
% Based on 2000 Calorie Diet	
Per Serving	% Daily Value
Calories 259	15.4%
Calories from fat 128	
Total Fat 14.2 g	22%
Saturated Fat 4.4g	22%
Cholesterol 365mg	122%
Sodium 1192mg	50%
Potassium 543mg	16%
Carbohydrates 4.5g	2%
Dietary Fiber 0.8g	3%
Sugars 2.4g	
Protein 27.3g	
Vitamin A 23%	Vitamin C 15%
Calcium 7%	Iron 14%

Eggs Your Way

1 Serving

Prep time: 5 min

Cook time: 10 min

Total time: 15 min

Sometimes simple is the best.

Ingredients:

- 2 eggs
- 1 tbsp. olive oil
- ¼ cup homemade salsa (p. 112)

Instructions:

1. Cook your eggs your favorite way. Scrambled, over easy, poached, whatever.
2. Smother in salsa.
3. Enjoy!

Nutrition Facts	
Serving Size 1 Serving	
% Based on 2000 Calorie Diet	
Per Serving	% Daily Value
Calories 281	14.0%
Calories from fat 207	
Total Fat 23.0 g	35%
Saturated Fat 4.8g	24%
Cholesterol 327mg	109%
Sodium 903mg	38%
Potassium 504mg	14%
Carbohydrates 8.8g	3%
Dietary Fiber 2.1g	8%

Sugars 4.7g	
Protein 13.1g	
Vitamin A 16%	Vitamin C 4%
Calcium 8%	Iron 12%

Lunches

Leftover Salad

Serves: 1
Prep time: 10 min
Total time: 10 min

Turn leftover protein into a tasty lunch!

Ingredients:
- 2 cups leafy greens of your choice
- 1 cup leftover protein, like chicken, pork or salmon. (Or 1 can of tuna fish).
- 1 oz. nuts or seeds
- 1/2 cup chopped fresh berries or other fruit of your choice
- 2 tbsp. Vinaigrette Dressing (p. 118)

Instructions:
1. Wash and dry the greens. Toast the nuts if you desire in an oven at 350, checking them every 2 minutes.
2. Place the greens in your serving dish. Top with your protein (I like to heat mine in the microwave first). Add the fruit and nuts. Dress, toss, and eat.

Nutrition Facts	
Serving Size 1 Serving	
% Based on 2000 Calorie Diet	
Per Serving	% Daily Value
Calories 605	30.25%
Calories from fat 314	
Total Fat 34.9g	54%
Saturated Fat 5.2g	26%

Cholesterol 108mg	36%
Sodium 150mg	6%
Potassium 1026mg	29%
Carbohydrates 18.5g	6%
Dietary Fiber 9.0g	9.0%
Sugars 5.5g	
Protein 51.1g	
Vitamin A 1%	Vitamin C 71%
Calcium 11%	Iron 14%

Pesto Egg Salad Wraps

Serves: 2
Prep time: 10 min
Total time: 10 min

An easy make-ahead lunch to take to work.

Ingredients:
- 3 hard-boiled eggs
- 1/3 c walnut basil pesto (p. 108)
- 1 celery stalk diced
- 4 large green lettuce or collard leaves

Instructions:
1. Wash and dry the lettuce leaves.
2. Peel the hard-boiled eggs and mash them with the pesto and celery. Spoon into the leaves and roll like a burrito.

Nutrition Facts	
Serving Size 1 Serving	
% Based on 2000 Calorie Diet	
Per Serving	% Daily Value
Calories 274	13.7%
Calories from fat 215	
Total Fat 23.9g	37%
Saturated Fat 5.4g	27%
Cholesterol 256mg	85%

Sodium 346mg	14%
Potassium 88mg	3%
Carbohydrates 3.2g	1%
Dietary Fiber 0.7g	3%
Sugars 3.2g	
Protein 12.3g	
Vitamin A 12%	Vitamin C 0%
Calcium 17%	Iron 8%

Turkey Wraps

Serves: 6
Prep time: 10 min
Total time: 10 min

A yummy sandwich without the bread!

Ingredients
1. 1 cucumber sliced
2. 2 Roma tomatoes sliced
3. 6 oz. sliced turkey lunch meat
4. 1/2 cup guacamole (p. 106)

Instructions:
Lay each turkey slice flat, and spread guacamole on it, like you would spread butter on bread. Lay the tomato and cucumber rounds on top of the avocado, and roll the turkey so all the goodness stays inside.

Nutrition Facts	
Serving Size 1 Serving	
% Based on 2000 Calorie Diet	
Per Serving	% Daily Value
Calories 487	24.35%
Calories from fat 195	
Total Fat 21.7g	33%
Saturated Fat 3.6g	18%
Cholesterol 82mg	27%
Sodium 1844mg	77%
Potassium 1340mg	38%
Carbohydrates 41.5g	14%
Dietary Fiber 11.0g	44%

Sugars 21.3g	
Protein 38.4g	
Vitamin A 60%	Vitamin C 150%
Calcium 6%	Iron 15%

Spicy Tuna Rolls

Serves: 1
Prep time: 10 min
Total time: 10 min

These tuna rolls are inspired by sushi but made in your kitchen. You can mix the tuna in advance, but don't roll in the seaweed until you are ready to eat, as it will get soggy.

Ingredients:
- 1 can tuna
- 1 tsp wasabi powder
- 1 tbsp. olive oil
- ½ cucumber julienned
- ½ avocado sliced
- 1 pack seaweed sheets

Instructions:
1. In a bowl, combine the tuna, olive oil, and wasabi powder.
2. Lay a seaweed sheet flat, and place a few cucumber spears and a slice of avocado on it.
3. Top with the tuna mixture, and roll up.

Nutrition Facts	
Serving Size 1 Serving	
% Based on 2000 Calorie Diet	
Per Serving	**% Daily Value**
Calories 564	28.2%
Calories from fat 321	
Total Fat 35.6g	55%
Saturated Fat 6.6g	33%

Cholesterol 50mg		17%	
Sodium 167mg		7%	
Potassium 1100mg		31%	
Carbohydrates 16.1g		5%	
Dietary Fiber 8.0g		32%	
Sugars 3.0g			
Protein 46.0g			
Vitamin A 10%		Vitamin C 32%	
Calcium 5%		Iron 20%	

Lemon Basil Chicken

Serves 6
Prep time: 25 min
Cook time: 75 min
Total time: 2 hours

This is one my son's favorite meals. Serve it with a green vegetable and drizzle the amazing sauce on your veggies. You can marinate the chicken ahead of time for a faster weeknight prep. You need the chicken skin for the unxious sauce, so don't remove it or substitute skinless breasts.

This sauce also works great with fish and vegetarian protein options, but reduce the amount of lemon juice you use by ½ to 3/4, or double the olive oil.

Ingredients
- 1 whole roasting or baking chicken
- 1/3 c olive oil
- 5 lemons
- 3 tbsp. fresh basil
- 5 cloves garlic
- Salt and pepper

Instructions:
Preheat oven to 400.

1. Cut up the chicken. If you've never cut up a chicken before, don't be intimidated! You can find great demonstrations on YouTube. Save the backbone and any organs for stock. (I throw them in the freezer until

a cold day when I want to warm my house with stock making.)

2. Squeeze the lemons until you have roughly 1/3 cup lemon juice.

3. Combine the olive oil and lemon juice. Press or mince the garlic cloves. Finely chop the basil and add it.* Add salt and pepper to taste.

4. Marinate the chicken in the lemon juice mixture for at least 15 minutes, but up to 24 hours.

5. Move the chicken and all of the marinade to a baking dish, and cook for 75 minutes or until done, turning the meat after the first 30 minutes.**

6. Serve with your favorite green vegetable.

Nutrition Facts Serving Size 1 Serving % Based on 2000 Calorie Diet	
Per Serving	% Daily Value
Calories 569	28.45%
Calories from fat 236	
Total Fat 26.2 g	40%
Saturated Fat 4.7g	23%
Cholesterol 228mg	76%
Sodium 261mg	11%
Potassium 676mg	19%
Carbohydrates 1.1g	0%
Dietary Fiber 0g	0%
Sugars 0g	
Protein 79.4g	
Vitamin A 3%	Vitamin C 12%
Calcium 5%	Iron 18%

* Cook's note: If you don't have a kitchen garden, buying fresh herbs can be expensive, and they often go bad if you don't use the whole package immediately. I like to buy the tubes of herbs in oil in the produce department and keep them in the fridge. It is a fast way to get fresh ginger, lemongrass, garlic, basil, dill, and lots of other flavors. If you use dried herbs, use only 1/3 the amount.

**This works well in a crock pot too. Brown the chicken pieces first for looks (or not if you don't care or have the time), and cook on low 8 hours, or high for 5.

Almond Chicken Fingers

Serves: 4

Prep time: 20 min

Cook time: 18 min

Total time: 48 min

You'll never notice there is no flour, and neither will your kids. If you like things spicy, add some cayenne into the coating.

A twist on this recipe is to make a vegetarian version by slicing tofu, freezing it for three days, and then bringing it back to room temperature and squeezing out the excess liquid. Use it in place of the chicken.

Ingredients:
- 1 cup almond meal or flour
- 1 lb. boneless, skinless chicken
- 2 eggs
- 2 tsp garlic salt
- 1 tbsp. Italian seasoning
- 1 tsp paprika
- Olive oil cooking spray or olive oil

Instructions:
1. Preheat oven to 400 F. Lightly grease a cookie sheet with olive oil.
2. Slice the chicken breasts into fingers.
3. Crack the eggs into a shallow bowl and lightly beat.
4. In another shallow bowl, add the almond meal and the spices and combine.
5. Dredge each chicken finger through the eggs, and then the almond flour mixture. Put on the baking sheet.

6. Bake the chicken for 6 minutes on each side. Then crank up your broiler to high, and broil for 3 minutes each side to make them crispy.

7. Serve with your favorite green vegetable.

Nutrition Facts	
Serving Size 1 Serving	
% Based on 2000 Calorie Diet	
Per Serving	% Daily Value
Calories 359	17.95%
Calories from fat 194	
Total Fat 21.6 g	33%
Saturated Fat 3.1g	15%
Cholesterol 157mg	52%
Sodium 93mg	4%
Potassium 411mg	12%
Carbohydrates 7.0g	2%
Dietary Fiber 3.3g	13%
Sugars 1.9g	
Protein 35.6g	
Vitamin A 8%	Vitamin C 1%
Calcium 9%	Iron 13%

Catfish Soup

Serves: 4
Prep time: 5 min
Cook time: 20 min
Total time: 25 min

This recipe is quick, easy, and oh so good! When my son was little, he called it "FishCat Soup." I often add shrimp or scallops along with the catfish if I'm making a double batch. You can substitute any white fish or shellfish, or even tofu (If you are vegetarian, you also need to substitute soy sauce for the fish sauce). If you are worried about the fat or sodium, you can substitute reduced fat coconut milk for the full-fat version, and low sodium soy sauce for the fish sauce.

Ingredients
- 2 cups vegetable stock or fish stock
- 2 tablespoons fresh lemongrass*
- 1 tbsp. minced ginger
- 1 tbsp. minced fresh cilantro
- ¼ cup fish sauce
- 4 limes
- 1 lb. catfish
- 1 14 oz. can coconut milk

Instructions:
1. In a large saucepan or small stockpot, heat the vegetable or fish stock to boiling over medium heat.
2. Juice the limes. You need about a ¼ cup.
3. Cut the fish into bite-sized pieces.
4. Once your stock is boiling, add the herbs, fish sauce, and lime juice to the pot and return to a boil.

5. Add the catfish and coconut milk. Simmer until the catfish is cooked, about five minutes. Ladle into bowls, and devour!

Nutrition Facts Serving Size 1 Serving % Based on 2000 Calorie Diet	
Per Serving	% Daily Value
Calories 507	25.35%
Calories from fat 351	
Total Fat 39.0 g	60%
Saturated Fat 24.7g	124%
Cholesterol 92mg	31%
Sodium 1773mg	74%
Potassium 735mg	21%
Carbohydrates 17.8g	6%
Dietary Fiber 3.7g	13%
Sugars 4.7g	
Protein 24.3g	
Vitamin A 1%	Vitamin C 5%
Calcium 8%	Iron 21%

*Chef's note – I buy tubes of lemongrass, minced ginger, and cilantro from the produce section for this recipe. This dish doesn't lend itself well to dried substitutes. If all you can find is dried lemongrass, steep it in the soup in a tea strainer, and then remove. Dried lemongrass has a very straw-like, unpleasant texture. Lemon zest would be a better substitute. If you haven't used fish sauce before, it is a liquefied anchovy paste. Look for it in the Asian aisle of the supermarket.

Baked Salmon

Serves: 4
Prep time: 5 min
Cook time: 15 min
Total time: 20 min

I have a confession: I prefer farm-raised salmon to wild. It is fattier and tastier to me. Fortunately, farm-raised salmon has come a long way in the past decade. The Monterey Bay Aquarium has a site/app called Seafood Watch that rates the best choices for fish. Check it out to find healthy, sustainable wild and farm-raised options.

Ingredients:
- 2 lbs. salmon filet
- 2 tsp dried oregano
- 2 tsp paprika
- 2 tsp garlic salt
- 1 tsp dried thyme
- 1 tsp black pepper
- Olive oil

Instructions
1. Preheat oven to 400 F. Brush a broiling pan with olive oil, and put the salmon, skin side down, in the pan. Brush the tops of the salmon filets with olive oil.
2. Combine all the spices in a small bowl, and sprinkle the mixture onto the salmon, coating the top evenly.
3. Bake at 400 for 15 minutes, or until the salmon in no longer raw in the center.
4. Serve with your favorite green vegetable.

Nutrition Facts

Serving Size 1 Serving % Based on 2000 Calorie Diet	
Per Serving	% Daily Value
Calories 321	16.05%
Calories from fat 191	
Total Fat 21.2 g	33%
Saturated Fat 3.1g	16%
Cholesterol 120mg	40%
Sodium 102mg	4%
Potassium 61mg	2%
Carbohydrates 2.6g	1%
Dietary Fiber 1.1g	4%
Sugars 0g	
Protein 44.7g	
Vitamin A 16%	Vitamin C 5%
Calcium 6%	Iron 14%

Roast Pork Tenderloin

Serves: 6
Prep time: 5 min
Cook time: 45 min
Total time: 1 hour

As a lean and tender meat dish, you can't beat pork tenderloin, and I have lots of recipes for fancy sauces. But I think it is also great without any accompaniment.

If you do want a sauce for your meat do the following:

Brown the pork first before roasting it. Then when you put it the oven, add two cups chicken stock. After the meat is cooked and is resting, scrape the bottom of the pan and boil down the remaining juices until it is the desired viscosity.

Ingredients:
- 1 2 lb. pork loin
- 4 tsp chopped fresh rosemary or 1 ½ tsp dried
- 4 garlic cloves minced or pressed, or 1 tbsp. of chopped garlic
- 1 tsp kosher salt
- 1/2 tsp pepper
- Olive oil

Instructions:
1. Preheat oven to 400 F.
2. Grease a small roasting pan with the olive oil.
3. Combine the herbs and spices and rub over the outside of the pork.
4. Roast about 45 minutes, or until the internal temperature of the meat is 145 F.

5. Let it rest for 10 minutes, slice in ½ in rounds, and serve with your favorite vegetables.

Nutrition Facts	
Serving Size 1 Serving	
% Based on 2000 Calorie Diet	
Per Serving	% Daily Value
Calories 392	39.2%
Calories from fat 212	
Total Fat 23.5 g	36%
Saturated Fat 8.3g	42%
Cholesterol 121mg	40%
Sodium 482mg	20%
Potassium 658mg	19%
Carbohydrates 1.3g	0%
Dietary Fiber 1.1g	4%
Sugars 0g	
Protein 41.5g	
Vitamin A 1%	Vitamin C 3%
Calcium 4%	Iron 9%

Pork 'Tacos'

Serves: 4
Prep time: 10 min
Cook time: 20 min
Total time: 30 min

This is a great way to use leftover roast pork tenderloin. Add pre-cooked meat at the last minute to just warm through.

Another twist is to simmer the tenderloin whole in a crockpot all day and shred the pork.

Or, substitute a meatless product, like tofu or crumbled tempeh.

Ingredients:
- 1 1 lb. pork tenderloin
- 1 tbsp. olive oil
- 1 small red onion
- 1 small jalapeno
- 1 bunch cilantro
- 1 lime
- ½ cup chicken broth
- 2 med tomatoes
- 2 medium avocados
- 1 head large lettuce leaves
- Salt and pepper to taste

Instructions:
1. Dice the onion and jalapeno.
2. Slice or cube the tenderloin and season with salt and pepper.
3. In a large skillet, heat the olive oil over med-low heat, and sauté the onion and jalapeño until soft, about 5

minutes. Crank the heat up to med-high, add the broth, the juice from the lime, and the pork.

4. Once the broth is boiling, reduce to a simmer, and leave uncovered, stirring occasionally until the pork is cooked through about 10 minutes. You want most of the liquid to evaporate.
5. While the pork is simmering, wash the lettuce leaves, chop the tomatoes, and slice the avocados.
6. Use the lettuce leaves for your tortillas, and top them with the pork mixture, tomatoes, and avocado slices.

Nutrition Facts	
Serving Size 1 Serving	
% Based on 2000 Calorie Diet	
Per Serving	% Daily Value
Calories 422	21.1%
Calories from fat 247	
Total Fat 27.5 g	42%
Saturated Fat 6.1g	30%
Cholesterol 83mg	28%
Sodium 173mg	7%
Potassium 1213mg	34%
Carbohydrates 15.0g	4%
Dietary Fiber 8.6g	32%
Sugars 3.4g	
Protein 33.2g	
Vitamin A 21%	Vitamin C 38%
Calcium 4%	Iron 13%

Buffaloaf

Serves 6
Prep time: 20 min
Cook time: 70 min
Total time: 1 hour, 40 min

Ground bison or buffalo is much leaner than ground beef. You can also substitute lean grass-fed beef if you prefer, or a meatless product.

Ingredients:
- 1 small yellow onion
- 2 celery ribs
- 1 carrot
- 3 garlic cloves
- 1/4 c water
- 2 large eggs
- 2 tablespoons tomato paste (no sugar added)
- 1 tablespoon Worcestershire sauce
- 1 tsp salt
- 1 tsp dried rosemary
- 1 tsp dried thyme
- ½ tsp ground black pepper
- 2 lbs. ground bison
- Olive oil

Instructions:
1. Preheat oven to 375 F. Grease a large roasting pan with olive oil.
2. Using a food processor or blender, puree the onion, celery, carrot, garlic, and water.

3. Heat a tablespoon of olive oil in a skillet over med-low heat. Sauté the vegetable mixture until the liquid has evaporated, roughly ten minutes.
4. Meanwhile, crack the eggs into a bowl, whisk lightly, add the tomato paste, Worcestershire sauce, salt, pepper, rosemary, thyme, and ground meat.
5. When the vegetables are ready, add them to the bowl, and stir just until combined.
6. Shape into a loaf, place in roasting pan, and cook for 70 minutes, or until a meat thermometer registers 160 F.
7. Let stand ten minutes, and serves with your favorite vegetables and homemade sugar-free ketchup (p. 116).

Nutrition Facts Serving Size 1 Serving % Based on 2000 Calorie Diet	
Per Serving	**% Daily Value**
Calories 403	20.15%
Calories from fat 222	
Total Fat 24.6 g	38%
Saturated Fat 10.3g	52%
Cholesterol 188mg	63%
Sodium 562mg	23%
Potassium 653mg	19%
Carbohydrates 4.6g	2%
Dietary Fiber 0.9	4%
Sugars 2.3g	
Protein 38.6g	
Vitamin A 38%	Vitamin C 6%
Calcium 5%	Iron 31%

Chimichurri Chicken Kabobs
Serves 4

A light, fun way to serve chicken. You can use this recipe with pork, steak, or a vegetarian alternative as well.

Ingredients:
+ 1 lb. boneless, skinless chicken breasts
+ 1 recipe Chimichurri sauce (p. 114)
+ 8 wooden skewers

Instructions:
1. Soak the skewers in water for 10 minutes.
2. Cut the chicken into large cubes, and marinate in ½ of the Chimichurri sauce.
3. Skewer the chicken and grill each side 2-3 minutes, until no longer pink inside.
4. Serve with your favorite vegetable, and the rest of the sauce for dipping.

Nutrition Facts	
Serving Size 1 Serving	
% Based on 2000 Calorie Diet	
Per Serving	% Daily Value
Calories 455	22.75%
Calories from fat 292	
Total Fat 32.4g	50%
Saturated Fat 3.9g	20%
Cholesterol 121mg	40%

Sodium 478mg	20%
Potassium 276mg	8%
Carbohydrates 4.0g	1%
Dietary Fiber 0g	0%
Sugars 0g	
Protein 33.6g	

Vitamin A 1%	Vitamin C 0%
Calcium 2%	Iron 8%

Roasted Vegetables

Serves: 6
Prep time: 5 min
Cook time: 30-45 min
Total time: 50 min

The great thing about this recipe is that it works for a variety of vegetables: broccoli, cauliflower, Brussels sprouts, etc. Experiment with different herbs and spices to change it up.

Ingredients:
- 2 lbs. broccoli, cauliflower, Brussel Sprouts, or a mixture
- 4 cloves garlic
- ¼ c olive oil
- 1 tsp salt

Instructions:
1. Preheat oven to 400 F.
2. Wash the vegetables and cut into bite size pieces. Spin them dry, removing as much water as possible.
3. Press the garlic and combine with the olive oil and salt.
4. Toss the veggies with the garlic mixture.
5. Turn after 20 minutes. Roast until cooked through, 30-45 minutes. (Note: Asparagus cooks in 3-5 minutes).

Nutrition Facts	
Serving Size 1 Serving	
% Based on 2000 Calorie Diet	
Per Serving	% Daily

	Value
Calories 126	6.3%
Calories from fat 80	
Total Fat 8.9g	14%
Saturated Fat 1.2g	6%
Cholesterol 0mg	0%
Sodium 438mg	18%
Potassium 487mg	14%
Carbohydrates 10.7g	4%
Dietary Fiber 4.0g	16%
Sugars 2.6g	
Protein 4.4g	
Vitamin A 19%	Vitamin C 226%
Calcium 7%	Iron 6%

Steamed Vegetables
Serves: 6
Prep time: 5 min
Cook time: 5-20 min
Total time: 25 min

This is another simple, tasty way to prepare a variety of veggies, including asparagus, green beans, broccoli, and cauliflower. Experiment with a variety of seasonings.

Ingredients:
- 2 lbs. vegetables of your choice
- 2 tbsp. Italian Seasonings
- 1 tsp. salt

Instructions:
1. Wash and trim vegetables.
2. Boil a large pot of water. When the bubbles are rolling, insert a steamer basket or colander into the top, not touching the top of the water. Place the veggies in the basket and cover with a lid. Steam until cooked to your liking, 5-20 minutes.
3. After the veggies are done, toss with the seasonings, and serve hot.

Nutrition Facts Serving Size 1 Serving % Based on 2000 Calorie Diet	
Per Serving	**% Daily Value**
Calories 66	3.3%

Calories from fat 17	
Total Fat 1.9g	3%
Saturated Fat 0g	0%
Cholesterol 3mg	1%
Sodium 439mg	18%
Potassium 481mg	14%
Carbohydrates 10.5g	4%
Dietary Fiber 3.9g	16%
Sugars 3.0g	
Protein 4.2g	
Vitamin A 19%	Vitamin C 225%
Calcium 7%	Iron 6%

Boiled Vegetables

Serves: 6
Prep time: 5 min
Cook time: 5-20 min
Total time: 25 min

Yet another way to prepare a variety of green vegetables. I like this preparation best with green beans.

Ingredients:

- 2 pounds green beans or another green vegetable
- 1/4 c olive oil
- Juice of 1 lemon

Instructions:

1. Wash and trim the vegetables as necessary.
2. Bring a large pot of water to a boil. Add the vegetables and cook until they are done to your liking, 3-10 minutes.
3. Drain in a large colander and return to the pot.
4. Toss with the olive oil and lemon juice. Serve hot.

Nutrition Facts	
Serving Size 1 Serving	
% Based on 2000 Calorie Diet	
Per Serving	% Daily Value
Calories 119	6.0%
Calories from fat 77	
Total Fat 8.6g	13%
Saturated Fat 1.2g	6%

Cholesterol 0mg	0%
Sodium 9mg	0%
Potassium 316mg	9%
Carbohydrates 10.8g	4%
Dietary Fiber 5.1g	21%
Sugars 2.1g	
Protein 2.8g	
Vitamin A 21%	Vitamin C 41%
Calcium 6%	Iron 9%

Sautéed Spinach with Salsa

Serves: 2
Cook time: 5 min
Total time: 7 min

Fast and so very flavorful. Try it with other leafy greens like kale and chard too.

Ingredients:
- 1 10 oz. bag of baby spinach (about 6 cups)
- 1/3 cup salsa (p. 112)
- 2 tbsp. olive oil

Instructions:
1. Wash and dry the spinach. In a large sauté pan, heat the oil over med-high heat. Wilt the spinach, stirring constantly, about five minutes.
2. Turn off the heat, and toss with the salsa. Serve immediately.

Nutrition Facts	
Serving Size 1 Serving	
% Based on 2000 Calorie Diet	
Per Serving	% Daily Value
Calories 142	7.1%
Calories from fat 127	
Total Fat 14.1g	13%
Saturated Fat 2.0g	10%
Cholesterol 0mg	0%

Sodium 315mg	13%
Potassium 129mg	4%
Carbohydrates 3.7g	1%
Dietary Fiber 0.7g	3%
Sugars 1.8g	
Protein 1.7g	
Vitamin A 58%	Vitamin C 6%
Calcium 4%	Iron 2%

Zoodles

Serves: 2
Prep time: 10 min
Cook time: 20 min
Total time: 30 min

Ingredients:

- 2 big zucchini
- ½ red onion sliced
- 1 pint cherry tomatoes
- 3 tbsp. olive oil
- 1/3 c pesto (p. 108)

Instructions:

1. Using a potato peeler or other tool designed for the job, peel the zucchini into long thin strips.
2. Slice the red onion.
3. Chop the cherry tomatoes in half.
4. Bring a large pot of water to a boil, and then add the zucchini. Boil for one minute, and then immerse in cold water to avoid overcooking.
5. In a pan, using 3 tbsp. olive oil over med-low heat, sauté the red onion until soft, about 10 minutes.
6. Add the cherry tomatoes and cook while constantly stirring for about 2 minutes.
7. Add the zoodles, mix and cook until you get a creamy mixture. Serve immediately.

Nutrition Facts	
Serving Size 1 Serving	
% Based on 2000 Calorie Diet	
Per Serving	% Daily Value
Calories 228	11.4%
Calories from fat 177	

Total Fat 19.6g	30%
Saturated Fat 3.3g	16%
Cholesterol 5mg	2%
Sodium 148mg	6%
Potassium 657mg	19%
Carbohydrates 11.5g	4%
Dietary Fiber 3.5g	14%
Sugars 7.1g	
Protein 4.9g	
Vitamin A 24%	Vitamin C 68%
Calcium 10%	Iron 5%

Fresh and Sweet "Orange" Juice

Serves: 1
Prep time: 10 min
Total time: 10 min

To satisfy a sugar craving.

Ingredients
- 2-3 large carrot sticks
- 1 celery stick
- ½ cup of seedless green grapes
- 1 cup water
- A sprinkling of fresh parsley

Instructions
1. Roughly chop up the carrots and celery.
2. Add the liquid base in the blender first.
3. Add the carrots and celery.
4. Add the grapes and parsley.
5. Blend at the highest speed for 30-45 seconds.

Nutrition Facts	
Serving Size 1 Serving	
% Based on 2000 Calorie Diet	
Per Serving	% Daily Value
Calories 168	8.4%
Calories from fat 7	
Total Fat 0.7g	1%
Saturated Fat 0g	0%

Cholesterol 0mg	0%
Sodium 172mg	7%
Potassium 799mg	23%
Carbohydrates 42.0g	14%
Dietary Fiber 6.9g	28%
Sugars 29.0g	
Protein 2.8g	

Vitamin A 837%	Vitamin C 43%
Calcium 10%	Iron 6%

Hummus

Serves: 3
Prep time: 10 min
Total time: 10 min

Experiment with different spices. Add cayenne pepper for some heat, or sundried tomatoes and basil.

Ingredients:
- 1 15 oz. can garbanzo beans
- 1 garlic clove
- Juice of 1 lemon
- ¼ cup roasted tahini
- ¼ c water
- 1 tbsp. extra virgin olive oil

Instructions:
1. Puree all ingredients in a food processor, adding more water if necessary.
2. Store in an airtight container in the refrigerator.

Nutrition Facts	
Serving Size 1 Serving	
% Based on 2000 Calorie Diet	
Per Serving	% Daily Value
Calories 288	14.4%
Calories from fat 162	
Total Fat 2.3g	28%
Saturated Fat 2.3g	12%

Cholesterol 0mg	0%
Sodium 311mg	13%
Potassium 4mg	0%
Carbohydrates 23.0g	8%
Dietary Fiber 6.6g	27%
Sugars 1.0g	
Protein 11.0g	
Vitamin A 2%	Vitamin C 6%
Calcium 7%	Iron 13%

Guacamole

Serves: 6
Prep time: 10 min
Total time: 10 min

Guacamole is a versatile, filling condiment that works great not just as a dip, but on sandwiches, eggs, vegetables, and meats.

Ingredients:

- 3 ripe avocados
- 1 jalapeno pepper
- Juice from 1 lime
- 1 tsp salt
- ¼ red onion
- 3 tbsp. chopped cilantro

Instructions:

1. Scoop the pulp from the avocado and place in a food processor.
2. Roughly chop the jalapeno and the stems from the cilantro, and add them to the food processor.
3. Add the other ingredients and puree. Adjust seasonings to taste.

Nutrition Facts Serving Size 1 Serving % Based on 2000 Calorie Diet	
Per Serving	% Daily Value
Calories 208	10.4%

Calories from fat 176	
Total Fat 19.6g	30%
Saturated Fat 4.1g	21%
Cholesterol 0mg	0%
Sodium 394mg	16%
Potassium 502mg	14%
Carbohydrates 9.2g	3%
Dietary Fiber 6.9g	28%
Sugars 0.8g	
Protein 2.0g	
Vitamin A 4%	Vitamin C 19%
Calcium 1%	Iron 4%

Walnut Basil Pesto

Serves: 6
Prep time: 10 min
Total time: 10 min

Another great versatile condiment to spice up anything!

Ingredients:
- 1 bunch basil
- ¾ cup extra virgin olive oil
- ½ c walnuts
- Juice of ½ lemon
- Salt to taste

Instructions:
1. Wash and dry the basil leaves.
2. Toast the walnuts either in a skillet or in a 350 oven, checking and stirring every minute to make sure they don't burn. Rub them with a paper towel to remove any black spots.
3. Place all ingredients in a food processor, and blend until smooth. Add olive oil if needed, and adjust seasonings.

Nutrition Facts Serving Size 1 Serving % Based on 2000 Calorie Diet	
Per Serving	% Daily

	Value
Calories 280	14.0%
Calories from fat 280	
Total Fat 31.4g	48%
Saturated Fat 4.0g	20%
Cholesterol 0mg	0%
Sodium 27mg	1%
Potassium 55mg	2%
Carbohydrates 1.0g	0%
Dietary Fiber 0.7g	3%
Sugars 2.1g	
Protein 2.5g	
Vitamin A 0%	Vitamin C 0%
Calcium 1%	Iron 2%

Homemade Nut butter

Serves: 8
Prep time: 20 min
Total time: 20 min

Ingredients:

- 2 cups raw nuts of your choice
- 2 tbsp. extra virgin olive oil
- ¼ tsp salt

Instructions:

1. First, roast the nuts in a 350 oven, checking and stirring every minute so they don't burn.
2. Rub the roasted nuts with a paper towel to remove any black spots.
3. Blend the nuts, oil, and salt in a food processor. Keep blending for up to 15 minutes, giving your food processor short breaks. The longer you blend, the more the nuts will release their oil and make a creamy butter.

Nutrition Facts	
Serving Size 1 Serving	
% Based on 2000 Calorie Diet	
Per Serving	% Daily Value
Calories 167	8.35%
Calories from fat 138	
Total Fat 15.4g	24%
Saturated Fat 1.4g	7%
Cholesterol 0mg	0%

Sodium 74mg	3%
Potassium 174mg	5%
Carbohydrates 5.1g	2%
Dietary Fiber 3.0g	12%
Sugars 1.0g	
Protein 5.0g	
Vitamin A 0%	Vitamin C 0%
Calcium 6%	Iron 0%

Homemade Pico de Gallo

Serves: 4
Prep time: 10 min
Total time: 10 min

If you've ever thought you've been blinded when you touched your eye hours after cutting chili peppers, you know that the liquid can remain on your hands and cause problems for quite a long time. Some people soak their hands in milk or yogurt after cutting chiles, and some people use gloves.

Ingredients:
- 1 lime
- 1 lb. fresh tomatoes (I use Roma)
- ½ red onion
- 1 jalapeno chile (use more or less per your preference)
- 1 bunch cilantro
- ¼ tsp dried oregano
- ¼ tsp cumin

Instructions:
1. Juice the lime.
2. Wash the vegetables and cilantro.
3. Roughly chop the tomatoes, onion, chiles. Roughly cut the leaves from the cilantro.
4. Put all ingredients in a food processor, and pulse to combine.
5. Store airtight in the fridge 3-5 days.

Nutrition Facts

Serving Size 1 Serving % Based on 2000 Calorie Diet	
Per Serving	% Daily Value
Calories 27	1.35%
Calories from fat 3	
Total Fat 0.3g	0%
Saturated Fat 0g	0%
Cholesterol 0mg	0%
Sodium 6mg	0%
Potassium 293mg	8%
Carbohydrates 5.8g	2%
Dietary Fiber 1.7g	7%
Sugars 2.1g	
Protein 1.2g	
Vitamin A 19%	Vitamin C 28%
Calcium 2%	Iron 3%

Chimichurri Sauce

Serves: 4
Prep time: 10 min
Total time: 10 min

This tangy sauce from Argentina is traditionally served with chicken or beef, but I love it on everything, from eggs to vegetables.

Ingredients:
- ½ c extra virgin olive oil
- 1/3 cup red wine vinegar
- ¼ cup packed fresh cilantro
- 1 cup packed fresh Italian parsley
- 6 large basil leaves
- 1 tsp crushed oregano, or 1/8 cup packed fresh leaves
- 4 garlic cloves
- ½ teaspoon ground cumin
- Salt and crushed red pepper to taste

Instructions:
1. Wash the herbs. Roughly remove the stems.
2. Peel the garlic.
3. Combine all ingredients in a food processor and puree.
4. Let it set for an hour at room temperature to combine flavors.

Nutrition Facts
Serving Size 1 Serving
% Based on 2000 Calorie Diet

Per Serving	% Daily Value
Calories 119	6.0%
Calories from fat 77	
Total Fat 8.6g	13%
Saturated Fat 1.2g	6%
Cholesterol 0mg	0%
Sodium 9mg	0%
Potassium 316mg	9%
Carbohydrates 10.8g	4%
Dietary Fiber 5.1g	21%
Sugars 2.1g	
Protein 2.8g	
Vitamin A 21%	Vitamin C 41%
Calcium 6%	Iron 9%

Simple Sugar-free ketchup

Makes: 1 ½ cups, 12 Servings
Serving Size: 2 tbsp.
Prep time: 10 min
Total time: 3 hours

If you are looking for a simple condiment for meatloaf or chicken fingers, here you go.

Ingredients:

- 1 6 oz. can tomato paste
- 2 tbsp. lemon juice
- ¼ tsp dry mustard
- 1/3 cup water
- ¼ tsp salt
- 1/4 tsp cinnamon
- A pinch ground cloves
- A pinch allspice
- A pinch cayenne pepper

Instructions:

Wisk all ingredients and refrigerate for 2-3 hours to combine the flavors.

Nutrition Facts	
Serving Size 1 Serving	
% Based on 2000 Calorie Diet	
Per Serving	% Daily Value
Calories 119	6.0%
Calories from fat 77	
Total Fat 8.6g	13%
Saturated Fat 1.2g	6%

Cholesterol 0mg		0%
Sodium 9mg		0%
Potassium 316mg		9%
Carbohydrates 10.8g		4%
Dietary Fiber 5.1g		21%
Sugars 2.1g		
Protein 2.8g		
Vitamin A 21%	Vitamin C 41%	
Calcium 6%	Iron 9%	

Vinaigrette Dressing

Serves: 8
Prep time: 10 min
Total time: 10 min

Experiment with different vinegars and herbs.

Ingredients:
- ½ c extra virgin olive oil
- 1/3 c vinegar of your choice
- 1 tbsp. minced garlic
- 1 tbsp. Italian seasoning

Instructions:

Mix all ingredients together and shake or whisk until well blended. Mix again before using.

Nutrition Facts	
Serving Size 1 Serving	
% Based on 2000 Calorie Diet	
Per Serving	% Daily Value
Calories 117	5.85%
Calories from fat 177	
Total Fat 13.1g	20%
Saturated Fat 1.9g	9%
Cholesterol 1mg	0%
Sodium 1mg	0%
Potassium 12mg	9%
Carbohydrates 0.6g	0%
Dietary Fiber 0g	0%
Sugars 2.1g	
Protein 0g	

Vitamin A 0%	Vitamin C 1%
Calcium 0%	Iron 0%

Conclusion

Too much sugar is a much bigger problem than most people realize.

Sugars are simple carbohydrates that are easy for the body to break down and use as energy. A little bit of sugar is vital for everyday functionality and health. Too much, (and anything more than a little is too much) can cause serious problems for your body. Too much sugar can disrupt the signals your brain uses to know when to consume calories and when to burn them. Too much sugar can also cause serious illnesses, such as diabetes and heart disease. Additionally, when consumed in excess, sugar is both physically and emotionally addictive.

There are many different forms of sugar, both 'natural' and 'processed', but they all break down into three monosaccharides called glucose, fructose, and galactose. Of the three, fructose tastes the sweetest. Fructose must be metabolized by the liver, and excess converts quickly to fat. Because High Fructose Corn Syrup is inexpensive to manufacture and easy to add to processed foods, its omnipresence has increased the general tolerance and expectation for sweet tastes in American food.

Far from helping the situation, artificial sugars compound the problem of too much sugar by increasing hypoglycemia and weight gain. Artificial sugars also come with a laundry list of other health concerns and do not provide any nutritional benefits.

In order to wean the body off of an excess of sugar without causing the brain to think it is starving, it is necessary to consume an adequate amount of lean protein and healthy fat, along with a moderate amount of sugar, ideally in the form of fruits that have fiber and micronutrients.

After ten days on a diet rich in lean protein and healthy fat and low in sugar, the body should have an easier time regulating the sugar and other calories it consumes.

Controlling sugar intake is critical for long-term health, and necessary for managing weight. It isn't especially easy, but it feels liberating to get control of sugar addiction.

I wish you the best of luck in following the 10-Day Sugar Detox, and congratulate you on taking control of your long-term health!

Message from the Author

Nothing tickles me more than when I hear from one of my readers. I love reading their stories of challenges and successes. Sometimes they even let me know when they find a typo in one of my books (for which am eternally grateful)! My writing is a work in progress. If there is something you think I can do to make this book a better experience for other readers, let me know about it. You can connect with me by email at francesca@brightideaseditoria.com, via twitter at @francescafoodie, or on my Facebook page.

If you'd like to help other readers decide if this book is for them, I'd be grateful if you could take a moment and post a sentence or two as a review on Amazon. Reader comments are the most powerful and unbiased way for others to determine which books should make the short list for their next read. And I promise I'll read every word.

Cheers,

Francesca

May I Suggest...

Other books by Francesca DiMarco

The 8 Day Green Smoothie Cleanse: Lose up to 13 Pounds in 8 Days with 25 Delicious Recipes

The Mediterranean Diet Cookbook for Beginners...who Love to Eat, with 75 Authentic Recipes by Executive Chef Kostas Magoulas

Other books published by Bright Ideas Editoria Ltd.
By Ryan J. S. Martin

Magnesium Deficiency: Weight Loss, Heart Disease and Depression, 13 Ways that Curing Your Magnesium Deficiency Can Rejuvenate Your Body

10,000 Steps: Walking for Weight Loss, Walking for Health: A Turn by Turn Roadmap

The Vitamin D Cure: 8 Surprising Ways Curing Your Vitamin D Deficiency Can Revitalize Your Health, Prevent Heart Disease and Cancer, and Help You Lose Weight

FREE DOWNLOAD

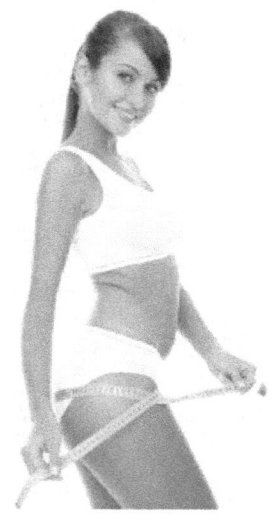

As a thank you for purchasing this book, I've created a free report full of weight loss hacks just for you!

TOP 10 WEIGHT LOSS HACKS - NO

DIETING ALLOWED!!!

"Free Report Reveals...The top 10 (ridiculously easy) weight loss hacks (Hint: You'll never believe #7)"

You can download the free report at
https://editoria.leadpages.co/weightlosshacks/

References

1 http://www.conncoll.edu/academics/internships-student-research/student-research-projects/are-oreos-addictive-nucleus-accumbens-c-fos-expression-is-correlated-with-conditioned-place-preference-to-cocaine-morphine-and-high-fatsugar-food-consumption.html

2 http://www.conncoll.edu/news/news-archive/2013/student-faculty-research-suggests-oreos-can-be-compared-to-drugs-of-abuse-in-lab-rats.html#.VVPMevlViko

3 http://www.livescience.com/40488-oreos-addictive-cocaine.html

4 http://www.ncbi.nlm.nih.gov/pmc/articles/PMC1931610/

5 http://addictions.about.com/od/aboutaddiction/a/Dsm-5-Criteria-For-Substance-Use-Disorders.htm

6 http://www.sciencedirect.com/science/article/pii/S0149763407000589

7 http://www.npr.org/sections/thesalt/2014/01/15/262741403/why-sugar-makes-us-feel-so-good

8 http://www.sucrose.com/lhist.html

9 http://www.medicaldaily.com/sugar-rush-stays-brains-memory-way-conserve-energy-later-322782

10 http://learn.fi.edu/learn/brain/carbs.html

11 http://www.webmd.com/diet/ss/slideshow-sugar-addiction

12 http://www.mynetdiary.com/carbs-in-weight-loss.html

13 http://health.howstuffworks.com/diseases-conditions/cardiovascular/cholesterol/foods-that-lower-cholesterol2.htm

14 http://www.livestrong.com/article/417962-how-does-the-body-digest-carbohydrates/

15 http://www.diabeteswellbeing.com/insulin-transfer-glucose-cells/

16 http://www.brainfacts.org/about-neuroscience/ask-an-expert/articles/2012/how-does-the-brain-use-food-as-energy/

17 http://www.endocrineweb.com/conditions/type-1-diabetes/what-insulin

18 http://www.news-medical.net/health/Lipogenesis-Control-and-Regulation.aspx

19 http://diabetes.niddk.nih.gov/dm/pubs/insulinresistance/#resistance

[20] http://www.ncbi.nlm.nih.gov/pubmed/3592616

[21] http://ajcn.nutrition.org/content/76/5/911.full

[22] http://www.sciencedaily.com/releases/1998/11/981126103305.htm

[23] http://www.cancercenter.com/discussions/blog/natural-vs-refined-sugars-whats-the-difference/

[24] http://www.bees-and-beekeeping.com/raw-honey-health-benefits.html

[25] http://www.webmd.com/diet/the-truth-about-agave

[26] http://www.webmd.com/diet/20080731/fructose-may-make-you-fatter

[27] http://www.statcan.gc.ca/pub/96-325-x/2007000/article/10576-eng.htm

[28] http://www.sugar.org/images/docs/refining-and-processing-sugar.pdf

[29] http://www.sugarindustrybiotechcouncil.org/sugar-beet-faq

[30] http://www.chow.com/food-news/54067/whats-the-difference-between-brown-sugars/

[31] http://askville.amazon.com/corn-syrup-invented-discovered-start-regular-basis-commercially/AnswerViewer.do?requestId=3834742

[32] http://en.wikipedia.org/wiki/High_fructose_corn_syrup

[33] http://www.eatingwell.com/nutrition_health/nutrition_news_information/is_high_fructose_corn_syrup_bad_for_you

[34] http://www.celestialhealing.net/Food_contain_HFCS.htm

[35] http://drhyman.com/blog/2011/05/13/5-reasons-high-fructose-corn-syrup-will-kill-you/#close

[36] http://www.foodpolitics.com/wp-content/uploads/HFCS_Rats_10.pdf

[37] http://sweetsurprise.com/princeton-study-on-obesity-and-hfcs

[38] http://examine.com/faq/is-hfcs-high-fructose-corn-syrup-worse-than-sugar.html/

[39] http://www.cancer.gov/about-cancer/causes-prevention/risk/diet/artificial-sweeteners-fact-sheet

[40] http://www.chemheritage.org/discover/media/magazine/articles/28-1-the-pursuit-of-sweet.aspx

[41] http://content.time.com/time/health/article/0,8599,1931116,00.html

[42] http://www.medicinenet.com/artificial_sweeteners/page5.htm

[43] http://dash.harvard.edu/bitstream/handle/1/8846759/Nill,_Ashley_-_The_History_of_Aspartame.pdf?sequence=3

[44] http://www.cancer.org/cancer/cancercauses/othercarcinogens/athome/aspartame

[45] http://dash.harvard.edu/bitstream/handle/1/8846759/Nill,_Ashley_-_The_History_of_Aspartame.pdf?sequence=3

[46] http://www.cspinet.org/reports/aspartame-Soffritti-EHP-2006.pdf

[47] ibid

[48] http://cspinet.org/reports/chemcuisine.htm#artificialsweeteners

[49] http://www.metric-conversions.org/weight/kilograms-to-pounds-table.htm

[50] http://www.theverge.com/2015/4/24/8489831/diet-pepsi-getting-rid-of-aspartame
[51] http://www.janethull.com/askdrhull/article.php?id=044
[52] http://www.theverge.com/2015/4/24/8489831/diet-pepsi-getting-rid-of-aspartame
[53] http://medical-dictionary.thefreedictionary.com/acetoacetic+acid
[54] http://www.referenceforbusiness.com/history2/22/Hoechst-A-G.html
[55] http://monsanto.unveiled.info/products/aspartme.htm
[56] http://www.sugar-and-sweetener-guide.com/acesulfameK.html
[57] http://juicingtherainbow.com/664/supermarket-juices/acesulfame-potassium-e950/
[58] https://www.cspinet.org/reports/chemcuisine.htm#acesulfamek
[59] http://www.kon.org/urc/frank.html
[60] http://en.wikipedia.org/wiki/Neotame
[61] http://www.sugar-and-sweetener-guide.com/neotame.html
[62] http://cspinet.org/reports/chemcuisine.htm#artificialsweeteners
[63] http://articles.mercola.com/sites/articles/archive/2012/03/28/neotame-more-toxic-than-aspartame.aspx
[64] https://www.cspinet.org/reports/chemcuisine.htm#advantame
[65] http://www.fda.gov/AboutFDA/Transparency/Basics/ucm214864.htm
[66] http://www.100daysofrealfood.com/2013/04/25/stevia-food-babe-investigates/
[67] http://www.livescience.com/39601-stevia-facts-safety.html
[68] http://cspinet.org/reports/chemcuisine.htm#stevia
[69] http://www.nature.com/nature/journal/v514/n7521/full/nature13793.html
[70] http://www.webmd.com/diet/20140917/artificial-sweeteners-blood-sugar?page=2
[71] http://www.the-scientist.com/?articles.view/articleNo/41033/title/Sugar-Substitutes--Gut-Bacteria--and-Glucose-Intolerance/
[72] http://theness.com/neurologicablog/index.php/artificial-sweeteners-and-diabetes/
[73] http://www.sciencedirect.com/science/article/pii/S0195666312004138
[74] http://www.ncbi.nlm.nih.gov/pubmed/23088901
[75] http://www.ncbi.nlm.nih.gov/pmc/articles/PMC2892765/
[76] http://articles.mercola.com/sites/articles/archive/2012/12/04/saccharin-aspartame-dangers.aspx#_edn5
[77] http://drhyman.com/blog/2010/06/19/artificial-sweeteners-could-be-sabotaging-your-diet/
[78] http://articles.mercola.com/sites/articles/archive/2014/01/05/dr-johnson-leptin-resistance.aspx
[79] http://www.webmd.com/diet/obesity/the-facts-on-leptin-faq?page=4
[80] http://www.ncbi.nlm.nih.gov/pmc/articles/PMC2584858/?tool=pmcentrez

[81] http://authoritynutrition.com/leptin-101/

[82] http://www.drkaslow.com/html/leptin_and_amylose.html

[83] http://www.healthambition.com/hormones-and-weight-loss-grhelin-leptin-lose-weight/

[84] http://nutritionwonderland.com/2010/05/understanding-our-bodies-insulin/

[85] http://drhyman.com/blog/2014/03/06/top-10-big-ideas-detox-sugar/

[86] http://www.health.harvard.edu/staying-healthy/the-truth-about-fats-bad-and-good

[87] https://evolvinghealth.wordpress.com/2013/05/22/is-it-time-to-stop-blaming-insulin-for-fat-storage/

[88] http://www.webmd.com/diet/sleep-and-weight-loss

[89] http://authoritynutrition.com/how-many-eggs-should-you-eat/

www.ingramcontent.com/pod-product-compliance
Lightning Source LLC
Chambersburg PA
CBHW060406290526
45791CB00002B/627